Light on Schizophrenia

Revealing causes and solutions
from an orthomolecular perspective

Abram Hoffer, MD, PhD

With contributions from

James Greenblatt, MD
Jonathan Prousky, ND, MSc
Paul Demeda, CNP

Light on Schizophrenia
Copyright © 2020 by The International Society for Orthomolecular Medicine

All rights reserved. No part of this publication may be reproduced, distributed, or transmitted in any form or by any means, including photocopying, recording, or other electronic or mechanical methods, without the prior written permission of The International Society for Orthomolecular Medicine, except in the case of brief quotations embodied in critical reviews and certain other non-commercial uses permitted by copyright law.

It is recommended that treatment of all health concerns be undertaken in consultation with a qualified health care professional.

This book should not be regarded as a substitute for professional medical advice.

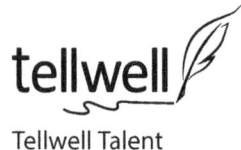

Tellwell Talent
www.tellwell.ca

ISBN
978-0-2288-3556-1 (Paperback)
978-0-2288-3557-8 (eBook)

Cover art by Dušan Petričić, commissioned for the Abram Hoffer Memorial Poster in 2009.

About this book...

This publication is an update to Dr. Abram Hoffer's book *Orthomolecular Treatment for Schizophrenia and other Mental Illness, A Guide for Practitioners*, originally published in 2007. Its purpose is to support and validate Dr. Hoffer's work, and add information that he might write about if he were alive today.

Dr. James Greenblatt and Dr. Jonathan Prousky have provided content segments for this update. Both doctors have extensive knowledge and clinical experience, acquired from many years of research and work with schizophrenia patients. Their contributions are invaluable additions to this publication.

This book is meant to be a useful introduction and resource for understanding schizophrenia from an orthomolecular perspective.

Much of the content of the original book is included in this update. To keep the legacy of Dr. Hoffer's original writing, the text of his original book exists alongside the updated content and is displayed in a contrasting typeface.

Dr. Hoffer's writing looks like this:

The original content is displayed throughout the book in this typeface.

Updated content looks like this:

The additional content from the various contributors is displayed in this typeface.

Table of contents

Preface 1

Introduction 4

Contributing factors for schizophrenia 9
Adrenochrome 9
Allergic or sensitivity reactions 9
Celiac disease and gluten sensitivity 11
Gliadorphin and casomorphin 16
Glutathione insufficiency 17
Histadelia 17
Histapenia 19
Homocysteine 19
Hypothyroid 20
Kynurenine pathway 23
Oxidative stress and inflammation ... 23
Pyroluria 24
The microbiome and the gut-brain axis 27
Toxic Metals 30

Modulators of schizophrenia 38
Niacin 39
Vitamin B6 (pyridoxine) 46
Vitamin C (ascorbic acid) 47
Vitamin D 49
Folate (folic acid) 50
Vitamin B12 52
Lithium 54
Magnesium 54
Zinc 55
Essential fatty acids 56
Amino acids 57
Medications 59

Orthomolecular treatment for Schizophrenia 66

Expanding Hoffer's orthomolecular treatment of schizophrenia 68
Schizophrenia psychosis and the tranquilizer psychosis 68
Recovery is possible with integrative orthomolecular treatment 69
Amino acid therapies 70
Broad-spectrum micronutrient treatment 73
Hormonal therapies 74
Improving the current situation 77
Putting it all together 77
In conclusion 78

Legacy chapter 81
Common questions about schizophrenia treatment 81
Relapses and orthomolecular therapy 82
Orthomolecular treatment for other mental illnesses 84

Conclusion 91

Biographies 92
Dr. Abram Hoffer 92
Dr. James Greenblatt 96
Dr. Jonathan Prousky 97
Paul Demeda 98

Acknowledgements 99

Preface

James Greenblatt, MD
Medical Director, Psychiatry Redefined Chief Medical Officer, Walden Behavioral Care

Schizophrenia may be the most complex, mysterious, and misunderstood psychiatric condition that has perplexed and frustrated clinicians over the past several decades. Despite ongoing research and efforts to improve its definition, diagnosis, and treatment, schizophrenia retains a stubborn presence in society.

Most recently defined in the Diagnostic and Statistical Manual of Mental Disorders (DSM-V) as a chronic disorder characterized by visual and auditory hallucinations, cognitive deficits, delusional beliefs, incoherent speech, and inappropriate behavior, schizophrenia can arise abruptly or gradually (McCutcheon, Marques, & Howes, 2019).

The World Health Organization currently estimates that schizophrenia affects at least 23 million individuals worldwide, representing a prevalence rate of roughly 1%. In addition to a higher incidence in young adults, statistics also indicate that schizophrenia occurs more often in men and is associated with ethnic, racial, and economic minorities. The latter evidence suggests a strong psychosocial contribution to the etiology and prognosis of the disease (World Health Organization, 2019).

Interestingly, cultural interpretations of schizophrenia symptoms differ widely, to the extent that the global prevalence rate is likely much higher (Morrill, 2017). Many developing societies assign theocentric or supernatural responsibility for mental illness, either exalting or ostracizing those with Western-defined schizophrenia symptoms. Some psychologists and philosophers have even proposed that schizophrenia is an advancement in evolutionary human biology, a theory that has gained favor among some genetic researchers (Scarr, Udawela, & Dean, 2018).

Beyond taxing medical systems, schizophrenia brings untold costs to prisons and homeless shelters, where hundreds of thousands go undiagnosed and lack proper care (Torrey, Zdanowicz, & Kennard, 2014).

In addition to a 5 to 10% greater risk of death by suicide, individuals with schizophrenia face a significantly shorter life expectancy, estimated at double to triple the risk of early death compared to typical American adults (McCutcheon, 2019).

The conventional treatment of schizophrenia has relied almost exclusively on an array of antipsychotic medications that offer moderate control of symptoms in some patients but deliver debilitating side effects in many (Chien & Yip, 2013).

Whether through ignorance, apathy, or arrogance, it is clear that the medical system has failed schizophrenia patients. Beyond unproductive diagnoses and ineffective treatments, most clinicians have neglected to comprehend the full picture of care needed to address the physical, psychological, functional, and sociological ramifications of schizophrenia, and support recovery of the patient as a whole person.

Without ignoring its biological aspects, schizophrenia is clearly a disease of socioeconomics: mounting data strongly link low income status at birth with lifetime risk of schizophrenia, a relationship strengthened by enduring poverty and chronic stress (Hakulinen, Webb, Pedersen, Agerbo, & Mok, 2019).

Notwithstanding the degree of knowledge, effort, and persistence required, patients deserve better, especially when multiple underexplored and underutilized treatment approaches exist.

Dr. Abram Hoffer's chief contributions to orthomolecular psychiatry began in 1952 when he performed the first double-blind therapeutic trials treating schizophrenia patients with high-dose niacin, after recognizing the remarkable similarities between psychosis and the neurological symptoms of pellagra.

Through his experiments with high-dose vitamin therapy, Hoffer demonstrated dramatic improvements in recovery and discharge rates in schizophrenia patients. Furthermore, he exhibited a holistic model of ethical care, removing sources of physical and emotional stress by providing comfortable shelter, adequate nourishment, and personal respect to each patient.

Hoffer's prolific career produced over five hundred scientific papers, two dozen books, and numerous collaborations with like-minded renegade experts, working tirelessly until the end of his life to leave a clear and imitable legacy worthy of more than a second glance.

A paragon of scientific inquiry, Hoffer searched existing information, compared and questioned data, developed and tested new hypotheses, reported honest results, and adjusted his views and theories according to new discoveries.

Furthermore, Hoffer never denied that antipsychotic medications were often necessary and effective when used appropriately and moderately, only emphasizing that pharmacotherapy should be one aspect rather than the entirety of treatment. Regardless, his experimental methods and clinical practices were repeatedly called into question and rejected by the medical establishment. The American Psychiatric Association and National Library of Medicine deliberately ostracized Hoffer and dismissed his research and case histories as non-"evidence-based medicine", publishing opposing data based on dissimilar and irrelevant study designs in patients with severe, irreversible damage.

Hoffer was ahead of his time in developing a biological model of a mental disorder, but arguably his greatest contribution is the example he set for doing whatever he could to find the answers needed to improve the treatment of schizophrenia patients and maintained hope that their lives could be better.

Hoffer's goal with each patient was complete recovery, including the absence of symptoms, familial and social harmony, and productive contribution to society (Hoffer, 2007). He was willing to exercise patience and accept small improvements as successful progress toward these goals.

Though he did not arrive at all of the answers in his lifetime, he set forth multiple testable hypotheses for others to build upon; indeed, to this day Hoffer's theories remain topics of research (Pires-Minard, 2017).

As Hoffer would attest, optimal mental health is not merely the absence of disease, but comprises both a healthy mind and body, autonomy, resilience, and a sense of happiness and fulfillment. Consequently, the integrative care model must address each of these areas from personal, familial, social, and environmental perspectives.

The information in this book is the product of one man's commitment to making a difference in patient's lives: a story every clinician needs to read, study, and benefit from the hope and encouragement found within Hoffer's words and in each patient's testimony.

References

Chien, W. T., & Yip, A. L. (2013). Current approaches to treatments for schizophrenia spectrum disorders, part I: an overview and medical treatments. *Neuropsychiatric Disease and Treatment, 9*, 1311.

Hakulinen, C., Webb, R. T., Pedersen, C. B., Agerbo, E., & Mok, P. L. (2019). Association between parental income during childhood and risk of schizophrenia later in life. *JAMA Psychiatry*.

Hoffer, A. (2007). *Orthomolecular treatment for schizophrenia and other mental ilnesses: A guide for practitioners*. International Schizophrenia Foundation.

McCutcheon, R. A., Marques, T. R., & Howes, O. D. (2019). Schizophrenia—An overview. *JAMA Psychiatry*, 1-10.

Morrill, Z. (2017). *Psychologists push for new approaches to psychosis: Part 1*. Mad In America website. https://www.madinamerica.com/2017/10/psychologists-push-new-approach-psychosis-part-1/. Accessed 11 Jan 2020.

Pires-Minard, A. (2017). *Is niacin a possible successful treatment for schizophrenia?* McGill University Office for Science and Society. https://www.mcgill.ca/oss/article/drugs-health-history-you-asked/niacin-possible-successful-treatment-schizophrenia. Accessed 28 Dec 2019.

Scarr, E., Udawela, M., & Dean, B. (2018). Changed frontal pole gene expression suggest altered interplay between neurotransmitter, developmental, and inflammatory pathways in schizophrenia. *NPJ Schizophrenia, 4*(1), 4.

Torrey, E. F., Zdanowicz, M. T., & Kennard, A. D. (2014). *The treatment of persons with mental illness in prisons and jails: A state survey*. Arlington, Va, Treatment Advocacy Center.

World Health Organization. (2019). *Schizophrenia*. https://www.who.int/news-room/fact-sheets/detail/schizophrenia. Accessed 28 Dec 2019.

Introduction

Abram Hoffer, MD

This guide is a resource for health practitioners who are interested in obtaining better results treating their patients and hope to start using the program.

It is also written for patients and their families who are not satisfied with the results they are seeing when only drugs are used and want to try a treatment which is ultimately safer and more effective.

The students who have mastered the material in this manual should be able to start successful treatment for mentally ill patients. As they continue to work with this approach they will become more and more enthusiastic and gradually expand their use of nutrients.

Most often medication is essential but orthomolecular physicians use drugs in optimum doses. When the drugs are combined with the orthomolecular approach, the amount of drug needed is much less and this decreases the incidence and the intensity of their side effects.

I will discuss the important aspects of treatment from nutrition including the role of allergies, the role of toxic foods, the role of diets too rich in refined carbohydrates, the role of a few key vitamins and minerals most often used, and the role of the essential fatty acids.

We are just at the beginning of major development in orthomolecular treatment. This guide is not meant to be a Bible or a cook book. It is not "writ in stone". It is a framework that practitioners can use in order to get started but each practitioner will add or subtract what is appropriate based upon their own experience in treatment and with each patient.

As more biochemical information accrues, more specific forms of the disease will be found and, with the appropriate laboratory tests, much more specific treatment will be available. There is no reason to think that the vitamins listed in this guide are the only ones.

A large amount of clinical material was published in the medical literature beginning with our first publication in 1957. The study was financed by the Government of Canada. We published originally in the establishment press until this information was suppressed by the combined efforts of the American Psychiatric Association and National Institute of Mental Health and others. We were forced to rely on our own journals, the *Journal of Orthomolecular Medicine* and its forerunners and in journals which deal with natural healing. These journals are becoming increasingly popular.

Medline consistently has refused to cover our journal for the past 33 years even though it covers *Time* magazine. Until the internet arrived this was a very effective way of censoring information that did not appeal to NIH.

Orthomolecular treatment

Orthomolecular is the term used by Linus Pauling to describe treatment that uses substances and molecules, that are normally present in the body. These are vitamins, minerals, essential fatty acids, amino acids, enzymes, and other substances normally present in food.

Nutrient dependency

A dependency is present when the need for any nutrient is so great that even what would be considered an optimum diet cannot provide the right amount.

This is due to genetic variation, to the vitamin-depleting effect of many drugs, to chronic mild deficiency, to increased need created by certain diseases, and to enzyme defects, so that important reactions in the body have to be driven by a greater quantity of that nutrient.

The term dependency was first used to describe patients who needed much larger amounts of vitamin B6. I have widened the meaning to apply to any condition and to any disease where large doses have been shown to be effective.

The first diseases that were recognized as deficiency diseases were beri beri, due to a deficiency of vitamin B1, scurvy, due to a deficiency of vitamin C, pellagra due to a deficiency of vitamin B3, and rickets due to a deficiency of vitamin D.

There are many other deficiencies but they are not characterized as readily. These diseases should be and usually are under control.

An extraordinary decision by the United States government during World War II forced the addition of vitamin B1, B2 and B3 to white flour. This logical decision eradicated pellagra which was one of the major scourges in the southeast United States and in some seasons helped fill their mental hospitals with psychotic pellagrins whose illness is identical with schizophrenia.

This enrichment of flour saved the United States billions of dollars in health costs and saved millions of people from the terrible ravages of this difficult but so easily preventable and treatable disease.

Phases of nutrient discovery

The history of the discovery of vitamins has gone through two phases. The first phase started about 1900. It led to the discovery of the vitamins, which was very important.

It also led to the RDAs which have proven to be very harmful when applied to every person. RDAs are recommended daily doses of vitamins which have become standard as if writ in holy stone.

This phase of vitamin theory and practice is called the vitamin–as-prevention paradigm. It is still with us, very powerful and is one of the main reasons why the use of large doses has been condemned. Its main principles are: (1) that vitamins are useful only to prevent classical deficiency diseases; (2) that vitamins must only be used in very small doses.

The second and currently developing phase is the vitamin-as-treatment phase. In this phase we recognize that there are other diseases that will respond to vitamins if used in optimum doses even though these conditions have not been recognized as vitamin dependencies.

Orthomolecular medicine deals primarily with optimum doses which may be very small as with vitamin B12 or very large as with vitamin B3 and vitamin C.

Schizophrenia treatment

The Saskatchewan research group, psychologists, psychiatrists, nurses, and social workers, all worked together under my direction when we introduced the use of vitamin B3 for treating the schizophrenias.

We conducted several prospective, randomized, double-blind controlled therapeutic trials starting in 1952 and we showed that adding the right amount of this vitamin to the treatment then available doubled the two-year schizophrenia recovery rate.

Since then many American and Canadian physicians corroborated our findings using the usual clinical open-ended methods. These methods are today considered merely anecdotal. Our original double-blind studies were, and still are ignored, as is the double-blind study by J. Richard Wittenborn who corroborated our findings working with a National Institute of Mental Health grant in New Jersey.

With the help of a small number of pioneer physicians, the treatment has been greatly expanded and we now use other nutrients as well, including vitamin C, the B-complex preparations which provide all the B vitamins, vitamin B6, folic acid, zinc, essential fatty acids and minerals.

What was originally a simple matter of giving our patients 1 g of vitamin B3 three times daily, in addition to whatever other treatment they were getting, has become much more sophisticated and much more efficacious.

Causes of schizophrenia

Schizophrenia is a syndrome not a disease. A syndrome is a constellation of symptoms and signs which may be caused by more than one factor.

Dr. Carl Pfeiffer was the first physician to clearly recognize the importance of the multiple causes of the schizophrenia syndrome. This is still not recognized in psychiatry where psychiatric diagnosis is entirely descriptive and not based upon clearly recognized causal factors. In his 1988 book *The Schizophrenias: Ours to Conquer*, he showed that schizophrenia causal factors can be divided into: pyroluria 30%; histadelia 20%; histapenia 50%; cerebral allergy 10%; wheat gluten allergy 4% and porphyria 0.1%.

The Quakers and modern schizophrenia treatment

About 150 years ago the Quakers in England developed the Moral Treatment of the Insane. The term schizophrenia had not been invented. The diagnostic term was insanity.

They reported a fifty percent recovery rate. Half of their patients recovered. They were really guests, not patients, since doctors and nurses were not involved. Dr. J Conolly, one of the foremost psychiatrists in England, reported the same recovery rate in his mental hospital. The Dorothea Dix Hospitals in New England at the same time also reported similar recovery rate. The recovery rate today, a century and a half later, is ten percent or less.

Decency and respect

The Quakers established houses, each housing 12 insane people. They were provided with shelter, with food, and they were treated with respect and decency. These three essential elements of any satisfactory treatment allowed their patients to heal.

Modern psychiatric hospitals do not treat their schizophrenic patients with decency and respect. Almost every one of the patients who are treated in these hospitals complain of the way they were treated.

The Quakers, in contrast, treated them as human beings. They would spend Saturday nights having dinner with them, and would interact and even dance with them. This is rare in most psychiatric wards although I suspect some of the very costly private hospitals might be somewhat better with this.

The natural recovery rate is facilitated by decreasing the patient's level of stress. Under stress the secretion of adrenalin in the body is increased. Adrenalin is the precursor of adrenochrome, one of the causes of psychosis. (Adrenochome will be discussed further on page 9)

Modern psychiatry does not provide proper shelter and too many patients subsist in grossly inadequate places including the streets of North American cities, under bridges, in parks, or in prison. This hardly qualifies as shelter and does nothing to alleviate stress. Too few patients are fortunate enough to have families that can provide adequate shelter.

The Quakers of 1850 had no access to modern food. They probably used the cheapest foods they could buy and that was, of course, advantageous, as it avoided antinutrients such as sugar and white flour.

Modern psychiatry does not show any interest in providing nourishing food for patients. Eat a few meals in any psychiatric ward and you'll see the food is too rich in refined carbohydrates, too poor in protein, too low in essential fatty acids and nearly devoid of essential nutrients.

The Quakers had no drugs and they did not use any of the harsh physical methods that were torture to the poor hapless patients in the usual mental hospitals of that day.

Modern xenobiotic psychiatry increases the stress on patients and obviously this is one explanation of their very low recovery rate. Xenobiotic compounds are substances that are not found naturally in living tissue.

Drugs do decrease the intensity of symptoms but do little to offer real recovery of a patient's former life. Bertrand Russell wrote "I believe four ingredients are necessary for happiness: health, warm personal relations, sufficient means to keep you from want, and successful work."

"Recovery" can mean something more than drugged docility, it can mean that patients are free of symptoms, that they are getting on well with their own family and with the community and that they are paying income tax or are otherwise productive in other activities.

Contributing factors for schizophrenia

Contributing factors are substances, contexts or conditions that have roles in the causation or promotion of schizophrenia.

Adrenochrome

Adrenochrome is a toxic derivative of adrenaline, which is thought to have a role in producing the psychotic features of schizophrenia.

The adrenal glands make adrenaline as part of the fight-or-flight response. When adrenaline is oxidized it becomes adrenolutin, which then creates adrenochrome.

People with schizophrenia can have a reduced capacity to degrade and remove adrenaline, and are therefore more susceptible to its negative effects, including the production of adrenochrome. However, the formation of adrenochrome, and its effects, can be influenced by nutrients like vitamin B3. (Adrenochrome is discussed further in the vitamin B3 section.)

Allergic or sensitivity reactions

There are two basic rules: to remove foods to which one is allergic and to remove foods which are toxic.

Allergic reactions may play a major role in almost every psychiatric syndrome, including mood disorders, schizophrenia, the anxiety states, children with learning and/or behavioral disorders.

Identifying allergies

One does not have to be an allergist but it does help to understand how one can quickly determine whether allergies are present. This is done by the history of allergic reactions beginning in infancy with colic which is usually a reaction to milk.

Common symptoms include; a history of many colds, runny noses, earaches, and tubes in the ears. Also these allergic children may display red ears, allergic shiners (as if they had not slept in ages) and suffer from chronic sinus congestion.

These may eventually clear but the body is still reactive. The symptoms change and the child develops behaviour and learning problems.

The allergic child may still have asthma, hay fever, rashes, and itches.

Often these patients love what they are allergic to and have great difficulty in eliminating these foods from their diet.

Very typical is a dislike of milk since it causes a lot of phlegm but a fondness for cheese, which is not so mucous forming. Yet cheese causes other symptoms such as gastrointestinal problems.

Patients are taught to look for a timing association between eating certain foods and the development of symptoms. If they get very sleepy one or two hours after a meal, i.e. lunch, they may be reacting adversely to one of the components of that meal.

Once a food is suspected it will finally be identified by an elimination diet which is more accurate than any skin or laboratory tests. The suspect food is eliminated for at least two weeks to one month. This is followed by the challenge test when that food is reintroduced.

If the patient is better when he is off the food and sick again when back on, a food allergy can be strongly suspected. The item is then avoided, often for life. Children suffer from fewer food allergies than adults. It gets worse with age.

The common ones for children are dairy products, sugar, eggs and wheat. For adults, allergens can be any food. The same procedure is used to identify foods that are toxic.

But even if there are no identifiable toxic foods, it is still a good idea to remove the free sugars. When these are eliminated it will also help to remove most of the other additives that are present in the diet.

Allergies and schizophrenia

There is a definite relationship between allergies and mental disorders including schizophrenias. But it is difficult for psychiatrists to accept this, since for a long time it has been taught that schizophrenic patients seldom have allergic reactions. This is mostly true if one ignores the reactions of their brain to the substances to which it is allergic. The term cerebral allergy has been used and the subject is covered by environmental medicine or clinical ecology.

Any chemical whether food, airborne or water born can cause reactions which maybe indistinguishable from the schizophrenic syndromes.

Every patient must be studied for the presence of these allergic reactions. The syndrome is schizophrenic and it may take any form. When these substances are eliminated it may take one to six months to become free of the effect of the foods patients have been allergic to for many years.

Allergic reactions can reproduce any one of the psychiatric disorders from children's learning and behavioral disorders, to anxiety and depression disorders, to the schizophrenic syndrome, to chronic fatigue states. Allergic reactions to sugar may be one of the main factors implicated in alcohol addiction.

A male alcoholic was admitted with severe delirium tremens. He was fasted for several days making sure his fluid intake was normal. When he recovered he was food-tested. The day he was given wheat in the morning, his wife complained bitterly that afternoon why had someone given him alcohol. He seemed disoriented from just the wheat. Anther day he was given potatoes. Shortly after that he had a grand mal convulsion. All addicts should be placed on diets that eliminate sugars.

Food allergies and fasting

About 40 years ago orthomolecular pioneers often got together to discuss their findings and to share ideas. We were mostly megavitamin therapists.

However two physicians, Dr. Marshall Mandell and Dr. William Philpott, began to tell us about the patients they had seen who became well when the foods they were reacting to were identified and removed from the diet. Allan Cott had visited Moscow for many weeks at their Institute for Chronic Schizophrenia to observe patients being treated by 30 day water fasts. They claimed that nearly two thirds got well.

This aroused my interest. About this time I was asked to make a house call because the patient was so rigid, catatonic, that she could not even sit up. I saw her and immediately called an ambulance. She agreed to fast.

To my surprise she was well after five days but she finished the fast and lost about 30 pounds in hospital. She then went back on foods using the Russian program but within a few days she was as sick as she had been on admission.

By this time I was aware of Mandell's and Philpott's work and concluded that the fast could be used as a way of determining what she was reacting to. After she had regained her weight she agreed to another fast but this time for only 5 days. Individual food testing proved that she was allergic to all meats. On a meat-free diet she was and remained normal.

First cases are very important, as they encourage further investigation. Over the next four to five years I fasted around 180 patients who had not responded well enough to my vitamin program. Ninety percent of the four-day water fasting was done at home. Of this group about 60% were much better at the end of the fast and the foods that made them ill was eliminated. It is most remarkable to see very psychotic patients recover by the end of a fast.

Celiac disease and gluten sensitivity

James Greenblatt, MD
Medical Director, Psychiatry Redefined

The term, "gluten" describes a pair of peptides inherent to wheat: gliadin and glutenin. With the addition of moisture and mixing, glutenin and gliadin combine to create the elastic gluten fibers that contribute to its utility in many foods. All cereal grains contain analogous peptides that can evoke similar digestive sensitivities.

Sensitivity and allergy

Epidemiological data indicate that roughly 1 in 7 Americans experience some unfavorable response to the ingestion of foods containing gluten, from identifiable gastrointestinal distress to nonspecific fatigue (Specter, 2014). Typical symptoms include abdominal pain, nausea, diarrhea, and constipation. Brain fog, mood changes, and muscle pain are also common. In the absence of adverse gastrointestinal reactions, extraintestinal symptoms are often missed or ignored.

A small percentage of the US population has a diagnosable food allergy to wheat, and similar to more prevalent allergies including peanuts, is associated with IgE antibodies against wheat (Specter, 2014). Mild allergic reactions to wheat trigger immediate, acute, and predictable symptoms such as swelling, hives, vomiting, or shortness of breath that quickly dissipate when the offender is removed; more severe reactions can induce anaphylaxis. Most damage is typically minimal and not widespread, allowing quick repair and restoration of normal function.

The majority of those reporting problems with gluten have no clinical indicators of allergy, and a new diagnosis of "non-Celiac gluten sensitivity" (NGCS) has recently emerged when symptoms appear in response to gluten but Celiac disease can be ruled out (Roszkowska, Pawlicka, Mroczek, Bałabuszek, & Nieradko-Iwanicka, 2019,).

Often mimicking irritable bowel syndrome and Crohn's disease, NGCS is often misdiagnosed by doctors and is commonly self-diagnosed, with some surveys reporting that one in three American adults avoid gluten.

Inflammation and leaky gut

When gluten is a persistent trigger, chronic inflammatory damage to intestinal tissue debilitates the epithelial layer separating the external world within the gastrointestinal tract from the body's internal environment, allowing foreign particles and organisms into systemic circulation that provoke an immune response throughout the body. Often referred to as "leaky gut", increased intestinal permeability is of growing interest to health experts across many disciplines (Bressan, & Kramer, 2016; Karakuła-Juchnowicz, Dzikowski, Pelczarska, Dzikowska, & Juchnowicz, 2016).

Autoimmunity

Although autoimmunity is not fully defined or understood, the etiologies of all autoimmune conditions share a similar framework: a genetic susceptibility and a triggering factor or event that activates a disproportionate immune response against healthy cells.

Interest in autoimmune disorders has expanded beyond gastroenterology, endocrinology, and rheumatology to include neurology and psychiatry.

Celiac disease

Definition, symptoms, and diagnosis

A typical Celiac symptom profile is similar to that of NGCS, although often more severe and accompanied by malnutrition and weight loss. At the same time, a substantial proportion of Celiac patients do not exhibit typical symptoms, experiencing skin conditions, neurological changes, or psychological abnormalities rather than gastrointestinal distress.

Today, at least 1% of the global population is officially diagnosed with Celiac disease, clinically defined by two key criteria. First, a positive serological test for autoantibodies to the tissue transglutaminase enzyme (tTG), a key enzyme involved in tissue repair and a unique autoimmune target in Celiac disease. Anti-endomysial antibodies (EMA) and anti-glutaminase (AGA) antibodies are also commonly assessed.

A confirmed diagnosis requires a biopsy of the intestinal tissue to evaluate the extent of damage to villi, and lymphocyte populations are often examined concurrently. Patients without evidence of intestinal damage are typically diagnosed with NCGS (Tye-Din, Galipeau, & Agardh, 2018).

Gluten, psychosis, and schizophrenia

Theories on the relationship

Decades of research have focused on psychosis and schizophrenia as some of the most severe manifestations of Celiac disease and gluten-sensitivity.

A recent comprehensive literature review of all available studies spotlighting the relationship between schizophrenia and gluten, reported that the majority of epidemiological, clinical, and case study evidence show a strong association, including measurable differences in immune and inflammatory makers, genotypes, and responses to a gluten-free diet (Dohan, 1973; Kalaydjian, Eaton, Cascella, & Fasano, 2006),

Similar inflammatory cytokine profiles among patients with gluten-sensitivity, Celiac disease, and schizophrenia emphasize the central role of chronic inflammation in each condition (Jeppesen & Benros, 2019). Today, roughly a quarter of Celiac patients experience comorbid neurological or psychiatric symptoms, and it has been estimated that Celiac patients have a five-fold risk of developing schizophrenia (Eaton et al., 2004; Kelly, et al., 2019). The most common neurological presentation in Celiac disease patients is ataxia resulting from inflammatory damage to central and peripheral nerves (Kalaydijan, 2006). Broader surveys indicate that half of individuals with a neurological condition may also have a gluten sensitivity.

At the most basic level, compromised integrity of the small intestine and impaired absorption often leads to nutrient deficiencies with broad implications for neural function and brain chemistry. A chronic pro-inflammatory state and autoimmune cascade activated by intestinal damage and increased gut permeability create collateral damage to other tissues, including the brain.

Secondary disease manifestations resulting from intestinal malabsorption and malnutrition offer a clear and undisputed mechanism linking gluten-sensitivity, Celiac, and schizophrenia. Deficiencies of iron, folate, and Vitamin B12 are frequently found in Celiac patients with profound consequences for cellular metabolism and turnover and for neurological function.

Insufficient zinc, copper, and Vitamin D are also common in Celiac and NGCS patients, each of which have been associated with schizophrenia pathology. In addition to maintaining normal homeostatic processes, these vitamins and minerals are essential for hormone production, neurotransmitter synthesis, and neural receptor function (Bledsoe et al., 2019); Roszkowska, 2019).

Gluten and neuroinflammation

Schizophrenia patients with a known gluten sensitivity have shown levels of key peripheral pro-inflammatory cytokines IL-1β and TNF-α twice as high as non-gluten-sensitive controls (Kelly et al., 2018). Significant positive correlations have also been reported between antibodies to gliadin and two neurochemicals associated with brain inflammation in a region of the brain previously linked to schizophrenia (Rowland et al., 2017). In each case, the data strongly suggest that gluten reactivity affects the brain as well, activating microglial immune cells and impairing neural function and regeneration (Nemani, Ghomi, McCormick, & Fan, 2015).

Physical and chemical brain abnormalities suggestive of neural death by recurring inflammation are present in both Celiac disease and schizophrenia, including cortical lesions and lower gray and white matter volumes (Ergün, Urhan, & Ayer, 2018).

Brain tissue loss reflects neural death, severing vital connections required for cell signaling and neurotransmitter synthesis (Buckley, 1998).

Auto-antibody comparisons in one of the most noteworthy studies into the association between schizophrenia and Celiac Disease, the 2011 Clinical Antipsychotic Trials of Intervention Effectiveness (CATIE), investigators noted that approximately 23% of schizophrenia patients had serological evidence of gluten sensitivity.

Zonulin

Zonulin, also known as pre-haptoglobin-2, is a recently discovered protein with functions that have profound implications for the gut-brain axis. First identified by Dr. Alessio Fasano in 1991, zonulin appears to be an exclusive regulator of epithelial tight junctions, having significant control over what passes from the intestinal lumen into systemic circulation. Intestinal epithelial cells and the tight junctions that connect them create a dynamic absorptive barrier and an intimate interplay with immune cells and the microbiome to maintain internal homeostasis (Bressan, 2016; Sturgeon & Fasano, 2016). In addition to specific bacteria, gliadin is one of the few currently known stimulators of zonulin release, implying that gluten induces an immune response analogous to several enterotoxic pathogens. Indeed, in vitro studies have demonstrated similar patterns of cytokine release by macrophages exposed to gliadin and bacteria (Sturgeon & Fasano, 2017).

Genomic studies have linked haptoglobin, the metabolic byproduct of zonulin, with several autoimmune, neurological, and psychiatric diseases including Celiac disease and schizophrenia, implying a common overexpression of zonulin as a result of shared genetic polymorphisms.

Zonulin offers not only a potential biomarker of inflammation but also a measurable status indicator of the gut-brain axis. Elevated serum zonulin resulting from a chronically breached intestinal barrier has recently been measured in the brain tissue of schizophrenia patients, suggesting zonulin's control over tight junctions may extend to the blood-brain barrier (Ergün et al., 2018). An influx of gluten antigens accelerates release of pro-inflammatory cytokines including IL-1β and TNF-α linked specifically to both Celiac and schizophrenia (Sturgeon & Fasano, 2017).

Fasano, zonulin's discoverer, once boldly proposed that Celiac patients with psychotic symptoms may frequently be misdiagnosed with schizophrenia.

Treatment avenues

Gluten-free diet

Although abundant studies demonstrate the psychiatric benefits of a gluten-free diet in Celiac patients, a survey of the evidence for treating schizophrenia patients with a gluten-free diet offers mixed outcomes (Ergün et al., 2018; Kalaydijan, 2006; Levinta, Mukovozov, & Tsoutsoulas, 2018).

On the other hand, it is not difficult to find striking case reports of complete and sustained symptom reversals emphasizing the profound gut-brain connection in susceptible schizophrenia patients (Delichatsios, 2016; De Santis, 1997).

Furthermore, some clinical support suggests that patients with gluten-compromised intestinal function and who require neuroleptic drugs, may improve on a gluten-free diet as a result of improved drug absorption (Ergün et al., 2018).

Biochemical individuality

At minimum, serum concentrations of IgA and IgG antibodies to glutaminase (AGA) and tissue transglutaminase (tTG) present a simple and reliable screening tool for identifying patients that may benefit from a gluten-free diet. Inflammatory markers including serum zonulin in combination with antibody data offer an additional layer of confidence. Urinary excretion levels of exorphins and genetic testing for a deficiency in the dipeptidyl peptidase-IV (DPP-IV) enzyme also highlight a subset of patients who may benefit from the withdrawal of gluten (Ergün et al., 2018). Tests for serum DPP-IV also have value as a clear and convenient marker of individual insufficiency to metabolize gluten peptides. Enzyme formulas with DPP-IV peptidase activity have become widely available as safe and effective therapeutic implements (Great Plains Laboratory, 2019).

Restoring GBA balance

Numerous dietary components and supplements enable healing of the intestinal barrier, support an inflammatory equilibrium, and encourage the growth of commensal bacteria.

Therapeutic treatment with high-dose probiotics is essential to increase the population of beneficial bacteria that modulate the inflammatory response, and facilitate bacterial synthesis of essential nutrients and hormones required for normal gut-brain communication. Research has also identified specific probiotic strains that may influence zonulin metabolism (Karakuła-Juchnowicz, 2016; Nemani et al., 2015).

Another critical step in rebalancing the GBA is reducing chronic inflammation and fostering an appropriate immune response to promote healing of damaged tissues. A well-rounded diet containing adequate protein, essential fatty acids, and antioxidants is key to providing the building blocks for cellular regeneration and neurotransmitter synthesis (Nemani et al., 2015)

Additionally, in most cases custom dietary supplement regimens target individual deficiencies and promote optimal brain chemistry including the B-vitamins, vitamin D, zinc, magnesium, and amino acids.

Gliadorphin and casomorphin

Gliadorphin and casomorphin are molecules generated from normal digestive breakdown of gluten and casein. Gliadorphin is derived from the gluten component of grains, and casomophin is derived from the casein component of dairy.

These molecules, classified as exorphins, have morphine-like properties (Ergün et al., 2018). They easily cross the blood-brain barrier and activate opiate receptors. At normal levels exorphins have roles in food-seeking and appetite regulation. At high levels they drive addictions and alter sensory perceptions (Pruimboom, & De Punder, 2015).

Other symptoms associated with high amounts of the exomorphins casomorphin and gliadorphin include speech and hearing problems; spaciness and "brain fog"; near-constant fatigue; irritability; aggression and moodiness; anxiety and depression; and sleep problems.

It has been reported that blood and urinary concentrations of exorphins from wheat and dairy are higher in schizophrenics (Bressan, & Kramer, 2016).

Causes of increased brain exorphins

Intestinal permeability

Increased intestinal permeability or "leaky gut" can allow large amounts of exorphins to enter the bloodstream from the digestive track and then access the brain.

DPP-IV insufficiency and exorphins

The enzyme DPP-IV has many physiological functions throughout the body. One of them is to break down gliadorphin and casomorphin to harmless amino acids.

The function of DPP-IV however, can be inhibited by the gliadin component of gluten. When DPP-IV is inhibited, less gliadorphin and casomorphin is broken down, so more of it reaches the brain. As well, with DPP-IV insufficiency other important roles of DPP-IV in the body, including endocrine and immune regulation, are compromised.

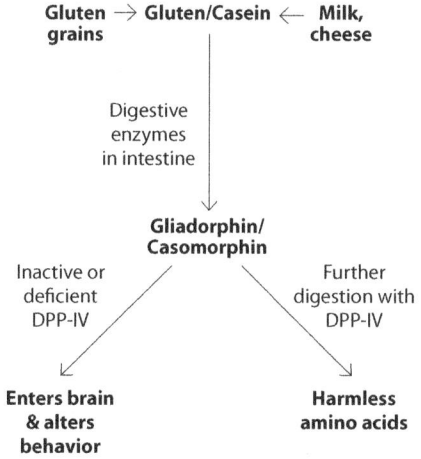

Gluten and Casein breakdown pathways

Drivers of DPP-IV insufficiency include overconsumption of wheat and milk, genetic susceptibility, antibiotics, gelatin from vaccines, *candida*, mercury and other heavy metals, pesticides, and nutritional deficiencies.

Glutathione insufficiency

Glutathione is a protective molecule in the body. Some of its roles include detoxification of free radicals and xenobiotics; maintenance of cellular thiols; and regeneration of vitamins C and E.

Glutathione and mental health

Insufficiency of glutathione is associated with multiple psychiatric and other physiological disorders, potentially as a result of the loss of glutathione's function in managing oxidative stress, mitochondrial disfunction, inflammation, as well as in glutamate and GABA regulation (Durieux, et al. 2015).

Glutathione levels in cerebrospinal fluid (CSF) and brain tissues of drug-naïve schizophrenia patients have been found to be 30–50% lower than controls. An inverse relationship between glutathione brain levels, cognitive and negative symptoms has been reported (Berk, et al. 2008; Phensy, et al., 2017).

Histadelia

Histadelia is a clinical syndrome that is promoted by elevated histamine levels.

Histadelic schizophrenic patients have too much histamine stored in basophils and mast cells.

In the presence of excess histamine, Dr. Pfeiffer described the histadelia syndrome as follows. Multiple allergies are commonly associated. Salivary secretion is increased so there is less tendency to suffer caries but gastric juices are increased which may lead to more heartburn. They often are compulsive high achievers but may suffer suicidal depression and become addicted easily.

The treatment Pfeiffer recommended included the following program:

- vitamin C 1 g twice daily,
- vitamin B6 dose increased until dream recall occurs,
- Dl methionine 500 to 1,000 mg twice daily,
- calcium 500 mg twice daily,
- zinc 10-30 mg daily,
- manganese 15-50 mg daily,
- Dilantin 100 mg twice daily,
- low protein diet to decrease the amount of the amino acid histidine from which histamine is derived, and
- avoid multivitamins and folic acid.

Pfeiffer did not recommend high doses of vitamin B3 and ascorbic acid and was very careful about using folic acid.

My experience has been different than Dr. Pfeiffer's. He is right when he recommends that histamine should be reduced but this can be achieved very well by the proper use of niacin. Niacin releases histamine from the storage cells. When these cells are examined with a microscope after the niacin flush, they show empty vesicles which had contained the histamine.

When I suspect high histamine levels in my schizophrenic patients I use the same procedure. But there are a few who cannot tolerate even tiny amounts and for them I use only niacinamide as a replacement.

I agree with Dr. Pfeiffer's classification but differ with him in the use of niacin. I have seen a few patients treated without B3 and they did not recover until niacin or niacinamide was added to their program.

The careful therapist will use whatever program helps patients. I think that one should start with the histadelic program and then add vitamin B3. Two grams of ascorbic acid is enough to mop up the histamine, which is released into the blood.

Vitamins B3, C and histadelia

The nicotinic acid form of vitamin B3 decreases tissue stores of histamine, which in turn helps lower blood levels. The nicotinamide form of vitamin B3 helps with histadelia by inhibiting mast cell histamine release.

Both the nicotinic acid and the nicotinamide forms of vitamin B3 may be required to address the nicotinamide adenine dinucleotide (NAD) deficiency that is considered the driver of histadelia.

Vitamin C has been shown to lower blood histamine levels. However people with schizophrenia may have impaired vitamin C metabolism, and a resulting increase in circulating histamine.

Suboticanec et al. found that schizophrenia patients had lower blood plasma vitamin C levels than controls, even though they had sufficient vitamin C intake from food (Suboticanec, Folnegović-Smalc, Korbar, Mestrović, & Buzina, 1990). This indicated that vitamin C supplementation may be required to address the effects of histadelia in schizophrenics.

Histamine and monoamine oxidase (MAO)

Histamine potentially binds the MAO enzyme, which promotes the oxidation of vitamin C instead of the inactivation dopamine. This would support the observation that schizophrenics tend to have reduced vitamin C and increased dopamine levels (Prousky 2007).

Histapenia

Histapenia is characterized by high blood copper and low histamine values. Excess copper may be the main reason. This is rather common due to copper and plastic plumbing.

In Vancouver, BC, with the soft water acidified by acid rain, the copper pipes are etched away so rapidly in some houses that they have to change their plumbing.

Copper destroys histamine. In Pfeiffer's unit the mean histamine level of a large number of histapenic patients was around 25 mcg/mL while normal levels are around 43 mcg/mL Copper levels were around 120 mg/mL. I prefer to see copper levels around 100 and zinc levels slightly higher than that.

When treated for histapenia, patients had the following time sequence of improvement. In the first month, sweaty palms, racing thoughts, insomnia and hypomania tend to diminish. By one year the hallucinations, obesity and paranoid ideas diminish.

The treatment Pfeiffer recommends included:
- high protein diet,
- vitamin B3 100-3,000 mg daily,
- folic acid 1-2 mg daily,
- zinc 10-30 mg daily,
- manganese 15-50 mg daily,
- lithium 300 to 900 mg daily,
- L-tryptophan 1,000 mg before bed,
- B12 injections 1 mg weekly,
- vitamin C 2 g daily, and
- molybdenum 500 mcg twice daily.

Homocysteine

Homocysteine is an amino acid that is made by the body and also supplied by food. Homocysteine levels are regulated by either of two major metabolic pathways. The re-methylation pathway converts homocysteine into methionine using vitamin B12 and folate. The trans-sulfuration pathway converts homocysteine into cysteine using vitamin B6.

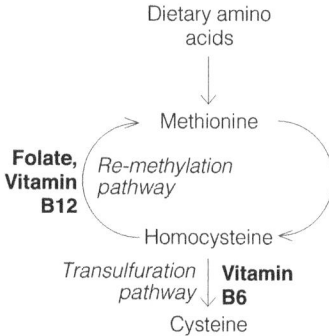

Homocysteine metabolism pathways and associated vitamins

Deficiencies of folate, vitamin B12, and vitamin B6 can result in increased homocysteine levels.

Elevated homocysteine levels are associated with mental issues including mild cognitive impairment, Alzheimer's Disease, Parkinson's Disease, depression, and schizophrenia (Kim & Moon. 2011)

Elevated homocysteine levels are found in some young male schizophrenic patients. Dr. R. Belmaker of Ben Gurion University, reported that schizophrenic patients given small amounts of folic acid, pyridoxine and B12 significantly reduced their symptoms after three months.

Hypothyroid

Schizophrenic patients can tolerate huge amounts of desiccated thyroid. Lewis Danziger in 1958 reported that every one of 80 schizophrenic who had been ill for six months or less recovered if they took between 120 and 1,200 mg daily for at least 100 days. If they stopped the thyroid they relapsed.

Soon after Danziger's first report appeared I gave a few of my patients desiccated thyroid. They were able to take an astonishing amount of thyroid without showing any clinical evidence of being overly stimulated by the hormone.

Harold Foster summarized the literature of the connection between schizophrenia and thyroid function. There is evidence that in the early phases there is too much thyroxine (T4) with no increase in triiodothyronine (T3). In the more chronic phases the amount of thyroid is reduced.

Foster suggests that the gland is damaged from chronic exposure to adrenochrome, a hallucinogen and powerful oxidant, and suggests that chronic patients who now need many years to recover might do so much more quickly if they were given adequate amounts of thyroid. I agree and prefer the desiccated form.

The thyroid stimulating hormone (TSH) test will not be very helpful: there is so much antagonism between thyroid specialists and others about depending upon the TSH, that it is difficult for physicians to give thyroid unless the fallible TSH is very low.

Thyroid hormones

The thyroid hormone thyroxine (T4) is created by the thyroid gland from tyrosine and iodine. Conversion of T4 into triiodothyronine (T3) occurs in the liver, kidneys, pituitary gland, and the nervous system. T3 binds to T3 receptors on cells to produce various metabolic effects.

Roles of thyroid hormones in healthy brain function

Thyroid hormones have important roles in brain health and function. They are mediators of neuronal cell migration, differentiation, signaling and brain maturation (Bernal, 2005). Thyroid hormones are also important for axonal outgrowth, dendritic branching and myelination (Calzà, Fernández & Giardino, 2015).

Thyroid hormones and neurotransmitters

Thyroid hormones affect the amount of dopamine receptors as well as the activity of the enzyme tyrosine hydroxylase (Santos et al., 2012). Tyrosine hydroxylase is required for the formation of dopamine, norepinephrine and epinephrine. Thyroid hormones also have roles in regulating serotonin and glutamate. (Santos et al., 2012)

The hypothyroid state

Hypothyroidism is a state of decreased effect of thyroid hormones on the body.

Common symptoms of hypothyroid include:
- cold intolerance,
- low body temperature,
- weakness,
- low energy or fatigue,
- easy weight gain,
- hair loss,
- pain,
- headache,
- PMS,
- insomnia,
- indigestion and constipation,
- elevated cholesterol, and
- frequent infections.

Mental symptoms of hypothyroid include (Pataracchia, 2008; Hoffer, 2001a):
- impaired cognition,
- anxiety or panic,
- depression,
- irritability, and
- poor memory or concentration.

Causes of hypothyroid

A low thyroid state can be caused by several factors including insufficient precursor molecules, autoimmune reactions, decreased production of T3, and T3 resistance.

Precursor molecules required for thyroid hormone production can be low due to low dietary intake. Analogous molecules like bromine and genistein, can compete with iodine and tyrosine for absorption and incorporation into thyroid hormones.

Autoimmune action against thyroid enzymes and TSH receptors reduce thyroid function.

Decreased conversion of T4 to the more metabolically active form T3 can result from (Hoffer, 2001a):
- stress,
- oxidative stress,
- environmental toxin exposures,
- liver and kidney issues,
- calorie restriction,
- sleep deprivation, and
- excessive exercise.

Thyroid hormone receptors on target cells can become resistant to T3 due to environmental toxins, as well as autoimmune, genetic and other factors.

Hypothyroid in the brain

Creation of T3 from T4 occurs in the brain, and requires sufficient amounts of T4 to cross the blood-cerebral spinal fluid barrier into the brain.

T4 is carried across the barrier by the transport protein transthyretin, however schizophrenics have been shown to have significantly lower CSF transthyretin. (Pataracchia, 2008)

Decreased transfer of T4 results in less active T3 in the brain, and less beneficial T3 metabolic activity. Conversion of T4 to T3 can be inhibited in the brain by cortisol. Cortisol levels in schizophrenics are often elevated, especially when they are experiencing stress.

Hypothyroid and schizophrenia

Hypothyroidism affects systems involved in schizophrenia including, metabolism of serotonin, dopamine, glutamate and GABA, as well as myelination and regulation of inflammation (Santos et al., 2012).

Deficiencies of thyroid hormone during brain development, and throughout life, can influence the manifestation of mental illness and response to its treatment (Santos et al., 2012).

Hypothyroidism is common in schizophrenia patients. (Santos et al., 2012). Low thyroid symptoms are often seen in patients with psychosis, moreover, schizophrenics can relapse when thyroid function is low. (Pataracchia, 2008)

Neonatal and infant thyroid hormone

The developing fetus relies on the mother for sufficient amounts of T4, so it is important to take into account the thyroid status of the mother during pregnancy (Santos et al., 2012).

Thyroid levels during neonatal and childhood development impact behaviour, locomotor ability, speech and cognition. Low amounts of thyroid hormone are associated with neuropsychological impairments (Santos et al., 2012).

Screening for hypothyroid

Research demonstrates the importance of screening patients with schizophrenia for abnormal thyroid status.

Abnormal thyroid hormone status with schizophrenia spectrum disorders

Serum thyroid hormones were reviewed from 343 patients admitted to an adult psychiatric unit. Tests included serum TSH, T4, T3, freeT4, free T3, and thyroid antibodies.

Abnormal thyroid results were seen in 29.3% of patients with schizophrenia-spectrum disorders, and 23.24 % of the patients with mood spectrum disorders (Radhakrishnan, Calvin, Singh, Thomas, & Srinivasan, 2013).

Thyroid testing approaches

Conventional TSH-only hormone testing may not reveal a low thyroid condition. The TSH test particularly correlates to the amount of T4 and not T3, whereas health and well-being are dependent on the availability of T3 (Hoffer, 2001a).

In a study by Skinner, published in 2000, 139 patients who where clinically hypothyroid had normal TSH values. When treated with T3 they recovered, demonstrating that TSH was not useful for revealing the T3 deficiency state (Hoffer, 2001a).

Testing a spectrum of thyroid related substances, like T4, T3, reverse T3, free T4 and T3, and thyroid antibodies can better illuminate thyroid status. Measurement of body temperature can be a simple way to reveal abnormal thyroid status.

Measuring T3 in urine may also be a useful indicator, as the results of a study examining 24-hour urine T3 in 832 patients concluded, "The determination of free T3 in the 24 hour urine has a far better correlation with the clinical thyroid status of a patient than any other classical test. The determination of free T3 in 24 hour urine collection provides a logical and practical answer to the many clinicians who are anxiously looking for laboratory confirmation of their clinical diagnosis in thyroid disease" (Baisier, Herloghe, & Eeckhaut, 2000).

Kynurenine pathway

The kynurenine pathway is a metabolic pathway that results in the production of NAD from the amino acid tryptophan.

The primary function of the pathway is to degrade tryptophan in order to, regulate tryptophan levels, deprive infectious organisms of tryptophan, and reduce autoimmune reactions.

Some kynurenine pathway metabolites contribute to schizophrenia symptoms. For example, kynurenic acid is an antagonist of CHRNA7 (nicotinic acetylcholine) and N-methyl-D-aspartate (NMDA) receptors. The metabolite 3-hydroxykynurenine has neurotoxic effects, and quinolinate is a neurotoxin and proconvulsant.

The kynurenine pathway initiated by the enzymes tryptophan 2,3 dioxygenase (TDO2) and by indolamine-2,3-dioxygenase (IDO). TDO2 activity is increased by tryptophan; low amounts of nicotinamide, niacin, and NAD; stress; and cortisol. IDO activity is increased by infections and inflammation.

Postmortem examination of brain tissue from schizophrenics has shown upregulation of TDO2 versus controls, and significant overproduction of kynurenine pathway intermediates (Prousky 2007).

An additional factor that is potentially implicated in upregulation of TDO2 is a reduced niacin effect—either due to low production of niacin, or issues with the niacin receptor (Prousky 2007).

Oxidative stress and inflammation

Evidence suggests that chronic oxidative stress and inflammation are contributors to multiple neuropsychiatric conditions (Joseph, Shukitt-Hale, Casadesus, & Fisher, 2005).

Oxidative stress, inflammation, and disease interact and promote ongoing negative effects.

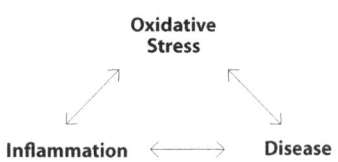

Interplay between oxidative stress, inflammation and disease

Oxidative stress

Oxidative stress occurs when free radical generation exceeds the neutralizing capacity of available antioxidants. Free radicals react with cell membranes, fatty acids, and proteins permanently reducing their functionality.

Internal sources of oxidative stress include metabolic processes, neurotransmitters, inflammatory responses, as well as infections and immune challenges.

External sources of oxidative stress include vitamin deficiencies, a high fat or sugar diet, environmental pollutants, drug abuse, stress, lack of exercise, and obesity.

Genetic variations (Single-nucleotide polymorphism (SNPs)) can also contribute to oxidative stress by altering enzymes related to metabolic rate, antioxidant and neurotransmitter function, and immune reactions.

Inflammation

Inflammation is a biological response to harmful stimuli, facilitated by immune cells and biochemicals.

Research shows connections between markers of inflammation and schizophrenia. For example, the cytokines IL-6 and IL-12 are implicated in negative symptoms of schizophrenia (Metcalf et al., 2017), and C-reactive protein (CRP) levels in adolescence are positively associated with schizophrenia in adulthood (Chase, Cone, Rosen, & Sharma, 2016; Crespo-Facorro et al., 2008).

Protective immune cells such as monocytes, B and T-cells, and dendritic cells show lower activity in schizophrenia patients (Fernandez-Egea et al., 2016).

Microglia are immune cells of the brain and CNS. Elevated microglia activity is a sign of infection or inflammatory processes and is correlated with high risk of schizophrenia (Bloomfield, et al., 2015).

Psychiatric illnesses associated with inflammation include depression, anxiety, bipolar disorder and schizophrenia (Salim, 2014).

Pyroluria

Pyroluria is a condition of overproduction of pyrroles. Pyrroles are a by-product of hemoglobin production and normally excreted in the urine.

Mauve factor is a pyrrole compound found in urine. It was mistakenly identified as kryptopyrrole, but is actually hydroxyhemopyrrolin-2-one (HPL). The terms "kryptopyrrole" and "HPL" are considered somewhat interchangeable.

Mauve factor was discovered in Saskatchewan in 1960. It was demonstrated by using long paper strips soaked in solution and allowing the solution and its contents to move up the paper by a wick action. Then they were dried and sprayed and the color developed. It stained mauve color and we called it the mauve factor. This method, called paper chromatography, is no longer used but was a well known method and earned the inventor, Dr. Tiselius, the Nobel prize.

When it was identified in collaboration with Carl Pfeiffer, the term mauve factor was changed to kryptopyrrole. They are similar but not identical.

Kryptopyrrole is a member of the pyrrole family, and may be correctly referred to as "urinary pyrrole".

Today this compound is being studied by many investigators especially in Europe. Dr. Woody McGinnis heads one such large study group. This substance appears to be a measure of oxidative stress.

Carl Pfeiffer developed a semi-quantitative test which is used to measure the amount of mauve factor in urine. It is found in up to 75% of schizophrenic patients depending upon how long they have been sick, and the treatment they have had. It is found in a very few healthy people under stress and is present in about one third of all non-psychotic patients no matter what the diagnosis is. About half of the children with infantile autism are positive.

In Saskatchewan the presence in urine was an indication to use vitamin B3 therapy no matter what these patients were called clinically.

Carl Pfeiffer showed that the mauve factor combined with pyridoxine and zinc to produce a double deficiency of pyridoxine and zinc. Therefore both of these nutrients were needed in the treatment program. Before this discovery, patients with this factor were treated in Saskatchewan as schizophrenic, mainly with vitamin B3. The addition of these two nutrients greatly improved the treatment results and decreased the need for as much vitamin B3.

If patient improved, the amount of kryptopyrrole went down to normal, very low levels. A relapse was usually preceded by a recurrence of the urinary factor.

Pyroluria: zinc and pyridoxine dependency

Pyroluria is the condition Osmond and I called malvaria (Hoffer & Osmond, 1963), i.e. patients who excrete too much "mauve factor." When this was identified, Pfeiffer called it pyroluria.

Clinically it is a schizophrenic syndrome but it has certain physical characteristics that often make it very easy to diagnose even without the urine test.

The presence of these signs are often very impressive to the patients and their parents. It helps convince them of a biochemical abnormality for which nutrients should be given.

Pfeiffer called it a deficiency but I believe it should more accurately called a dependency since the conditions inducing this mauve factor are not primarily due to a deficiency in the diet. Their needs are far above what any diet could provide.

McGinnis reviewed the current state of knowledge about the mauve factor (McGinnis, 2004a).

The qualitative assay available at the time revealed the so-called 'mauve Factor' in about two-thirds of recent-onset schizophrenics, but not in controls.

One hundred percent of the schizophrenic subgroup which recovered on high-dose niacinamide (vitamin B3) were found to have converted from mauve-positive to mauve-negative.

Relapses associated with discontinuation of niacinamide were associated with reappearance of mauve.

The signs of high amounts of kryptopyrrole are most prevalent in adolescents and children and include white areas in their fingernails, fragile nails, pain in the joints often the knees, lack of pigment in the skin, skin infections and acne, sometimes morning nausea, poor dream recall, insomnia and of course the psychiatric symptoms.

The usual treatment is used but should include adequate amounts of pyridoxine and zinc. I prescribe up to 250 mg of pyridoxine after each meal and up to 100 mg of zinc citrate daily. I have not seen any problems with these doses in over forty years.

Many women with severe premenstrual tension are pyroluriacs and often with the proper use of pyridoxine and zinc, the PMS will be gone in three months.

Mauve factor, stress, and oxidative stress

Higher urinary mauve values are associated with stress (many publications have confirmed this).

In both humans and animals, an ample body of research demonstrates that emotional, non-physically painful stress increases oxidative stress, measurable as actual oxidized biomolecules.

The behavioral and somatic disorders associated with higher urinary mauve are also associated with higher markers for oxidative stress.

B6 and zinc and B3 are powerful anti-oxidants, which supports the suggestion that mauve is associated with oxidative stress.

That seemingly disparate treatments, niacinamide on one hand, vitamin B6 and zinc on the other, decrease mauve and produce concomitant symptomatic improvement is intriguing.

Lower zinc, as found in higher-mauve states, certainly is associated with oxidative stress.

Dairy consumption and pyroluria

There is a frequent association between milk allergy and pyroluria. This is based upon the physical signs not on laboratory tests.

Dairy products do inhibit the absorption of zinc from the food.

Pyroluria and mental health

Mental symptoms of pyroluria are largely related to zinc and vitamin B6 deficiencies. Symptoms of these deficiencies include:
- poor short-term memory,
- poor stress control,
- severe inner tension,
- episodic anger,
- nervousness,
- anxiety and depression, and
- mood swings

Neurobehavioral disorders associated with elevated mauve factor (HPL)

Diagnosis	With elevated HPL (%)
Intermittent porphyria	100
Schizophrenia, acute	59-80
Schizophrenia, chronic	40-50
Criminal behavior	
Adults, sudden deviance	71
Youths, violent offenders	33
Bipolar Disorder	47-50
Depression	12-46
ADHD	40-47
Alcoholism	20-84

(McGinnis, 2004b)

Diagnosing pyroluria

Pyroluria can be objectively diagnosed by elevated levels of HPL, as measured by the kryptopyrrole quantitative urine test.

	Kryptopyrrole level
Optimal	0-10 mcg/dL
Borderline pyroluria	10-15 mcg/dL
Pyroluria	**> 15 mcg/dL**

(Greenblatt, 2018)

The amount of kryptopyrrole can fluctuate dramatically. Stress, illness, and injury increase levels. For optimal test results, urine should be collected during a period of increased stress.

Treating pyroluria

William Walsh, of the Pfeiffer Treatment Center, found that using treatment based upon biochemical markers, of which mauve factors was one, decreased frequency of assaultive behaviour significantly in 92% of the subjects treated and 58% achieved complete remission (Walsh, Glab, & Haakenson, 2004).

With mild to moderate pyroluria, treatment typically reduces HPL levels quickly. Severe pyroluria usually responds gradually over 3 to 12 months. Symptoms typically recur within 2 to 4 weeks if supplementation is stopped (McGinnis, 2004b).

Greenblatt (2018) recommended daily supplementation of 200-800 mg of vitamin B6 in the pyridoxal-5-phosphate form and 25–100 mg of zinc for addressing pyroluria.

Prousky (2006) stated in an article: "Although I could test for this compound, I choose not to, since these nutrients are inexpensive and have minimal side effects. The daily dosages I routinely start with are 250 mg of pyridoxine and 50 mg of zinc".

The microbiome and the gut-brain axis

James Greenblatt, MD
Medical Director, Psychiatry Redefined

The gut-brain axis

The gut-brain axis (GBA) is becoming well-characterized as the leading mechanism behind many neurological, mood, and behavioral disorders.

Encompassing the entire digestive tract and central nervous system, the GBA also incorporates the immune system and microbiome, representing a synergistic ecosystem.

Consequently, as the central regulator of the inflammatory and immune response, the gastrointestinal tract and GBA represent a key area of focus for elucidating the pathophysiology of schizophrenia (Ergün et al., 2018; Karakuła-Juchnowicz, Dzikowski, Pelczarska, Dzikowska, & Juchnowicz, 2016).

New genetic data have narrowed in on the intestinal barrier as the principal activation site for many autoimmune and psychiatric conditions. As part of the normal inflammatory response, intestinal permeability is increased to quickly mobilize immune cells to a site of injury or invasion. This process can end up doing more harm than good when chronic stimulation forces tight junctions between intestinal epithelial cells to remain open abnormally, not only allowing unwarranted influx of foreign particles but facilitating damage to the delicate inner intestinal layer.

By representing the multi-directional communication between the gastrointestinal tract, the immune system, and the brain, mediated through the central nervous system via hormones and neurotransmitters, the GBA drives thought, perception, and mood (Nemani et al., 2015).

In combination with immune-mediated neuroinflammatory damage, impediments to normal brain signaling and processing are behind the array of cognitive, sensory, and emotional distortions presented by schizophrenia patients.

As the intestinal barrier represents the principal site of the immune system, the composition and integrity of the microbiome inevitably influences the nature of its response. Intestinal dysbiosis often results from gut barrier disruption driven by a chronic immune response, contributing to imbalance of the gut-brain axis.

Multiple lines of evidence confirm that specific alterations are present in the microbiome of patients with Celiac disease and schizophrenia, and consensus supports a bidirectional influence (Ergün et al., 2018).

The microbiome's influence on the GBA may begin in early brain development through modulation of critical neural growth factors and neurotransmitter receptors specifically linked to symptoms of schizophrenia and other psychiatric disorders.

The role of intestinal microbiota on the brain is evidenced in part by the positive effect of probiotic therapy on psychiatric patients, including multiple studies with schizophrenia patients. Data suggest that beneficial bacteria modulate inflammation in the brain by dampening the immune response.

The microbiome may also promote the synthesis of brain-derived neurotropic factor (BDNF), a critical growth factor for neurons that is also involved in the function of NMDA neurotransmitter receptors, a well-established relationship found to be central in schizophrenia pathology ((Buckley, Pillai, & Howell, 2011; Maqsood & Stone, 2016; Nemani et al., 2015).

In Celiac disease, in addition to loss of normal barrier function, dysbiosis of the microbiome inhibits production of anti-inflammatory immune cells and cytokines that are necessary to bring immune reactions back into balance. Neuroimaging studies of chronic inflammation demonstrate that pro-inflammatory cytokines also activate microglia in the brain that encourage neuroinflammation and demyelination (Ergün et al., 2018; Nemani et al., 2015).

The gut-brain axis and mental health

Mental health conditions affected by the gut-brain axis include anxiety and depression, autism, obsessive compulsive disorder, and schizophrenia. Gut issues affected by the gut brain axis include dysbiosis, inflammation and appetite.

Schizophrenia and the microbiome

Assessment of the microbiome in the context of schizophrenia suggest that schizophrenia is associated with (Nguyen, Kosciolek, Eyler, Knight, & Jeste, 2018):
- reduced microbial diversity, and differences in community composition compared to controls,
- increased intestinal inflammation and permeability, and
- microbial populations that are associated with depressive and psychotic symptoms, compromised physical health and sleep.

Gut microbiome and remission with FEP

Schwarz et al. appraised gut microbiota in 28 patients with first-episode psychosis (FEP) and 16 controls, and assessed symptoms at baseline and 12 months post-treatment.

The FEP patients had different gut microbial composition than controls. The subgroup of patients with the worst dysbiosis experienced decreased global functioning, increased negative symptoms, and less frequent remission.

After 12 months, 70% of patients whose microbiota were similar to controls showed remission, while only 28% of patients with imbalanced microbiota showed remission (Schwarz et al. 2018).

Benefits of probiotics

Probiotics, BDNF, and immune regulation

Tomasik, Yolken, Bahn, & Dickerson, (2015) measured Immune-related serum proteins in patients before and after probiotic treatment.

The probiotics treatment increased levels of BDNF, and regulated immune and intestinal epithelial cells.

HPHPA

HPHPA is the abbreviation for 3-(3-hydroxyphenyl)-3- hydroxypropionic acid, which is a metabolite of anaerobic *Clostridium* bacteria in the gut. HPHPA has been shown to be elevated in urine samples from patients with schizophrenia (Shaw, 2010).

High levels of HPHPA are associated with behavioral, gastrointestinal, and neuropsychiatric issues.

HPHPA inactivates the enzyme dopamine beta hydroxylase, which can result in overproduction of dopamine, reduced levels of norepinephrine, and decreased glutathione production. These changes can promote abnormal or psychotic behaviour.

Addressing HPHPA

HPHPA levels in the gut can be assessed with organic acids testing.

Probiotic supplementation can help normalize gut flora as well as decrease HPHPA levels. *Clostridia*-specific antibiotics can be added if probiotics aren't effective in 2-3 months (Greenblatt, 2018).

Toxic metals

Toxic metals such as lead, mercury, and cadmium are pervasive in the environment. An abundance of research shows that the accumulation of these metals in the body has negative impacts on health.

The brain is especially susceptible to accumulation and storage of fat-soluble toxic metals because of its high fatty-acid composition (Orisakwe, 2014).

Toxic metals bind tissues, and interfere with the functions of essential minerals (Sears, 2018).

As well, the high level of metabolic activity of the brain and excessive oxidative stress caused by toxic metals, can promote free radical damage to important components and molecules in the brain.

Toxic metals compete with essential minerals for absorption and transportation, which means poor nutrition increases the risk for toxicity (Sears, 2018).

Toxic metals and mental health

Humans are highly vulnerable to neuropsychiatric diseases caused by exposures to toxic metals (Orisakwe, 2014).

Young children are especially at risk, as toxic metals affect early brain development, resulting in the potential for life-long intellectual and behavioural impairments (Sears, 2018). "The link between exposure to different metals and adverse early neurodevelopmental outcomes is well known" (Modabbernia et al., 2016).

Blood toxic metals higher and minerals lower in schizophrenia

In a study by Arinola, Idonije, Akinlade, & Ihenyen, (2010), blood levels of trace metals were analyzed in 35 schizophrenia patients who were either newly diagnosed but not taking antipsychotic drugs (APDs), or who were taking antipsychotic drugs for at least two weeks. Twenty healthy volunteers served as controls.

Compared to controls, levels of lead, chromium and cadmium were significantly higher in the newly diagnosed patients, and chromium and cadmium were higher in the patients taking medication. As well, the metal-countering minerals iron and selenium, were significantly lower in the schizophrenia patients than the controls.

Lead

Lead interferes with normal calcium metabolism, resulting in decreased neurotransmitter release at synapses, and spontaneous release of neurotransmitters in neurons that would not normally be involved in the intended mental process (Gearing, 2016).

Exposure to lead has been linked to under-functioning NMDA receptors, resulting in improper regulation of BDNF signaling and synaptic functioning (Modabbernia et al., 2016; Neal & Guilarte, 2010). Lead disrupts cellular energy production, and in developing brains, it negatively affects hippocampal neurons and glial cell function (Modabbernia et al., 2016).

Lead and mental health

Toxic levels of lead are associated with (Pataracchia, 2008):
- psychosis,
- behavioural issues,
- mood disorders,
- learning disabilities,
- insomnia,
- compromised immunity,
- brain damage,
- delayed infant development, and
- disruption of thyroid hormone transport into the brain.

Childhood lead exposure correlates with schizophrenia symptoms

Baby teeth from nine schizophrenic adults and five healthy adults were analyzed to determine the amount and timing of metal exposures during the critically important neurodevelopmental periods of early life. Exposures were then compared to later-life risk of schizophrenia.

Results showed that lead levels were higher in the baby teeth of schizophrenic patients. As well, early-life lead levels positively correlated with adult psychotic experiences, and negatively correlated with adult IQ. (Modabbernia et al., 2016)

Sources of lead include (Campbell, 1995):
- lead paint,
- drinking water,
- lead water pipes,
- leaded glass and pottery,
- newsprint,
- car batteries,
- organ meats,
- tobacco, and
- cosmetics.

Although now phased out, lead from leaded gas persists in the environment and continues to be a source lead-induced health effects. (Eschner, 2016).

Mercury

The brain is the main target organ for mercury in the body. It disrupts neurotransmitter function and normal brain protein metabolism. Mercury stimulates brain excitotoxins resulting in damage to brain tissue and peripheral nerves (Bernhoft, 2011).

Mercury can cross the placenta and be passed to newborns through breast milk. (Yang et al., 1997)

Sources of mercury include (Pataracchia, 2008; US EPA, OCSPP, 2020):
- fish and shellfish,
- dental fillings,
- vaccines,
- novelty jewelry,
- some skin products,
- thermometers, and
- fluorescent lights.

Aluminum

Aluminum is a neurotoxin that promotes neurodegeneration. Negative effects of aluminum on brain development include changes in neurotransmitter synthesis, axonal transport and synaptic transmission (Inan-Eroglu & Ayaz, 2018).

Cognition, learning, and memory are affected by aluminum and it has been shown to have toxic effects in schizophrenia patients (Pataracchia, 2008).

Sources of aluminum include (Pataracchia, 2008: Exley, 2013):
- aluminum cookware,
- drinking boxes,
- drinking water,
- processed cheese,
- antiperspirants,
- cosmetics,
- sunscreens,
- antacids and medications, and
- adjuvant in vaccines and allergy treatments.

Cadmium

Cell proliferation, differentiation, and apoptosis are negatively affected by cadmium. As well, cadmium impairs cellular energy production by inhibiting cellular respiration and oxidative phosphorylation.

Cadmium depletes protective glutathione, and binds sulfhydryl groups. It increases production of reactive oxygen species (ROS), and inhibits protective antioxidant enzymes. As well, cadmium may inhibit the enzyme monoamine oxidase to promote neurotransmitter imbalances (Rafati, Mehravar, Rahimzadeh, & Moghadamnia, 2017).

Attention, psychomotor activity, and memory are negatively affected by cadmium. Exposure during prenatal and neonatal periods has been shown to cause anxiety, mood disorders, and schizophrenia in later life. Increased cadmium levels have been reported in schizophrenia patients. (Orisakwe, 2014).

Sources of cadmium include:
- paint pigments,
- polyvinyl chloride plastic products,
- soft plastic toys,
- fossil fuel burning,
- contaminated food, and
- cigarette smoke.

Blood samples of cigarette smokers contained cadmium levels four to five times higher than non-smokers in one study (Rafati, Mehravar, Rahimzadeh, & Moghadamnia, 2017).

Copper

Copper is an essential mineral in human metabolism. However, in excess, it can be harmful to the body. Copper toxicity is very common in schizophrenia (Pataracchia, 2008).

Excess copper increases the production of damaging reactive oxygen species in the brain, as well as the oxidation of serotonin into potentially hallucinogenic molecules (Jones, Underwood, Coulson, & Taylor, 2007).

Copper also increases the conversion of dopamine to norepinephrine and epinephrine, which can promote feelings of anxiety, panic, and agitation (Tsafrir, 2017).

Sources of copper include (Pataracchia, 2008; Pfeiffer, 1974; Tsafrir, 2017):
- plant and animal foods which have been exposed to pesticides and fungicides or grown in contaminated soil,
- seafood from contaminated seawater areas,
- copper water piping,
- cigarette smoke, and
- oral contraceptive use.

Other contributors to excessive copper levels include zinc deficiency, and a low thyroid condition. With low thyroid function, production of the copper-regulating proteins metallothionein and ceruloplasmin is reduced (Pataracchia, 2008).

Arsenic

Arsenic exposure can result in neuropsychiatric outcomes including:
- impaired memory,
- agitation,
- disorientation,
- mania,
- dementia,
- emotional lability,
- frontal lobe dysfunction, and
- delirium, hallucinations, and psychosis.

Environmental sources of arsenic include (ATSDR, 2009):
- algaecides and herbicides,
- pressure-treated wood, and
- emissions from coal-fired power plants.

Food sources of arsenic include:
- foods grown in arsenic-contaminated soil;
- bottom dwelling or feeding seafoods, including clams, oysters, crabs, and lobsters;
- seaweed; and
- chicken and rice (Center for Veterinary Medicine 2019).

Manganese

Although manganese has essential functions in the brain, in excess it has neurotoxic effects. These effects are considered to be induced by oxidative stress, DNA damage, and mitochondrial dysfunction (Bornhorst, 2012).

In a study of 114 schizophrenics and 114 controls, higher manganese levels were associated with an increased risk of schizophrenia (Tiebing et al., 2015).

Symptoms of manganese toxicity include (Bornhorst et al., 2012; Roth, 2006):
- tiredness,
- behavioral and mood changes,
- intellectual deficits,
- compulsive behaviors, and
- dystonia.

Environmental manganese exposures include:
- manufacturing of textiles, leather, glass, and batteries;
- combustion of fossil fuels;
- agricultural fertilizer;
- pesticides; and
- some plant foods, especially wheat and rice, and tea leaves. (World Health Organization Regional Office for Europe Copenhagen, 2000).

Evaluating and addressing toxic metals

Assessing toxic metal accumulation

Assessing metal toxicity can be a complicated process. A logical starting point would be taking an extensive patient exposure history, so that current sources of toxins can be identified and avoided.

However, because patients often have poor recollection or are unaware of the sources of their exposure, the patient history may not be enough to accurately uncover exposures. Other ways to assess the presence of toxic metals include blood, urine, hair and nail testing.

Blood tests for toxic metals can show acute and immediate toxic metal exposure, while hair and nail testing can reveal exposures over the previous months.

Testing the accumulated body load of toxic metals can be done by testing urine after ingesting of a challenge molecule like dimercaptosuccinic acid (DMSA), or ethylenediaminetetraacetic acid (EDTA).

Endogenous mobilization of toxic metals

Toxic metals that have accumulated in soft tissues and bone over time, can be released back into body circulation, serving as a source of exposure even after the original external source has been removed. The mobilization of stored toxic metals from body tissues can result from trauma, pregnancy, menopause, extreme starvation, and severe emotional stress (Sears, 2018).

Addressing toxic metal accumulation

Environmental and dietary sources of toxic metal exposures need to be removed as much as possible.

Many patients will improve with a basic protocol of a healthy diet, supplementation of essential nutrients, exercise and rest. Sweating from exercise or sauna can also help remove toxic metals (Sears, 2018).

Detoxification of toxic metals must be properly supported with a protocol tailored to the patients unique situation and toxic load, in order to minimize the risk of releasing, then depositing the metals back into tissues. The best approach for brain detoxification is conservatively, "with repeated, modest treatments, using multiple agents" (Sears, 2018).

Considering the ubiquitous exposure to toxic metals in our modern world, and their effects on brain health, it makes sense to look at identifying and addressing these toxins in schizophrenia patients.

References

Arinola, G., Idonije, B., Akinlade, K., & Ihenyen, O. (2010). Essential trace metals and heavy metals in newly diagnosed schizophrenic patients and those on anti-psychotic medication. *Journal of Research in Medical Sciences: The Official Journal of Isfahan University of Medical Sciences, 15*(5), 245–249.

ATSDR. (2009). *Arsenic toxicity case study: where is arsenic found?* | ATSDR - Environmental Medicine & Environmental Health Education - CSEM. Environmental Health and Medicine Education. Retrieved April 30, 2020, from https://www.atsdr.cdc.gov/csem/csem.asp?csem=1&po=5.

Baisier, W. V., Hertoghe, J., & Eeckhaut, W. (2000). Thyroid insufficiency. Is TSH measurement the only diagnostic tool? *Journal of Nutritional & Environmental Medicine*, *10*(2), 105–113. doi: 10.1080/13590840050043521.

Berk, M., Copolov, D., Dean, O., Lu, K., Jeavons, S., Schapkaitz, I., ... & Ording-Jespersen, S. (2008). N-acetyl cysteine as a glutathione precursor for schizophrenia – a double-blind, randomized, placebo-controlled trial. *Biological Psychiatry*, *64*(5), 361-368.

Bernal, J. (2005). Thyroid hormones and brain development. *Vitamins & Hormones*, 95–122. doi: 10.1016/s0083-6729(05)71004-9.

Bernhoft, R. A. (2012). Mercury toxicity and treatment: A review of the literature. *Journal of Environmental and Public Health*, 2012. https://doi.org/10.1155/2012/460508.

Bledsoe, A. C., King, K. S., Larson, J. J., Snyder, M., Absah, I., Choung, R. S., & Murray, J. A. (2019). Micronutrient deficiencies are common in contemporary celiac disease despite lack of overt malabsorption symptoms. *Mayo Clinic Proceedings*, *94*(7), 1253–1260. https://doi.org/10.1016/j.mayocp.2018.11.036

Bloomfield, P. S., Selvaraj, S., Veronese, M., Rizzo, G., Bertoldo, A., Owen, D. R., ... Howes, O. D. (2016). Microglial activity in people at ultra high risk of psychosis and in schizophrenia: An [11C]PBR28 PET brain imaging study. *American Journal of Psychiatry*, *173*(1), 44–52. doi: 10.1176/appi.ajp.2015.14101358.

Bornhorst, J., Wehe, C. A., Hüwel, S., Karst, U., Galla, H.-J., & Schwerdtle, T. (2012). Impact of manganese on and transfer across blood-brain and blood-cerebrospinal fluid barrier in vitro. *Journal of Biological Chemistry*, *287*(21), 17140–17151. https://doi.org/10.1074/jbc.M112.344093.

Bressan, P., & Kramer, P. (2016). Bread and other edible agents of mental disease. *Frontiers in human neuroscience*, *10*, 130.

Buckley, P. F. (1998). Structural brain imaging in schizophrenia. *Psychiatric Clinics of North America*, *21*(1), 77-92.

Buckley, P. F., Pillai, A., & Howell, K. R. (2011). Brain-derived neurotrophic factor: findings in schizophrenia. *Current Opinion in Psychiatry*, *24*(2), 122-127.

Calzà, L., Fernández, M., & Giardino, L. (2015). Role of the thyroid system in myelination and neural connectivity. *Comprehensive Physiology*, *5*(3), 1405–1421. doi: 10.1002/cphy.c140035.

Campbell, D. (1995). Minerals and disease. *Journal of Orthomolecular Medicine*, *10*(3 & 4).

Center for Veterinary Medicine. (2019). *Arsenic-based animal drugs and poultry*. FDA. https://www.fda.gov/animal-veterinary/product-safety-information/arsenic-based-animal-drugs-and-poultry.

Chase, K. A., Cone, J. J., Rosen, C., & Sharma, R. P. (2016). The value of interleukin 6 as a peripheral diagnostic marker in schizophrenia. *BMC Psychiatry*, *16*(1), 152.

Crespo-Facorro, B., Carrasco-Marín, E., Pérez-Iglesias, R., Pelayo-Terán, J. M., Fernandez-Prieto, L., Leyva-Cobián, F., & Vázquez-Barquero, J. L. (2008). Interleukin-12 plasma levels in drug-naive patients with a first episode of psychosis: effects of antipsychotic drugs. *Psychiatry Research*, *158*(2), 206-216.

Dohan, F. C. (1973). Coeliac disease and schizophrenia. *British Medical Journal*, *3*(5870), 51.

Durieux, A. M. S., Fernandes, C., Murphy, D., Labouesse, M. A., Giovanoli, S., Meyer, U., Li, Q., So, P.-W., & McAlonan, G. (2015). Targeting glia with N-acetylcysteine modulates brain glutamate and behaviors relevant to neurodevelopmental disorders in C57BL/6J mice. *Frontiers in Behavioral Neuroscience*, *9*, 343. https://doi.org/10.3389/fnbeh.2015.00343.

Eaton, W., Mortensen, P. B., Agerbo, E., Byrne, M., Mors, O., & Ewald, H. (2004). Coeliac disease and schizophrenia: population based case control study with linkage of Danish national registers. *BMJ*, *328*(7437), 438-439.

Ergün, C., Urhan, M., & Ayer, A. (2018). A review on the relationship between gluten and schizophrenia: Is gluten the cause?. *Nutritional Neuroscience*, *21*(7), 455-466.

Eschner, K. (2016). *Leaded gas was a known poison the day it was invented*. Smithsonian Magazine. Retrieved May 4, 2020, from https://www.smithsonianmag.com/smart-news/leaded-gas-poison-invented-180961368/.

Exley, C. (2013). Human exposure to aluminium. *Environmental Science. Processes & Impacts*, *15*(10), 1807–1816. https://doi.org/10.1039/c3em00374d.

Fernandez-Egea, E., Vértes, P. E., Flint, S. M., Turner, L., Mustafa, S., Hatton, A., ... & Bullmore, E. T. (2016). Peripheral immune cell populations associated with cognitive deficits and negative symptoms of treatment-resistant schizophrenia. *PloS One*, *11*(5), e0155631.

Gearing, M. (2016). *The deadly biology of lead exposure—Science in the news*. Harvard University. Retrieved May 4, 2020, from http://sitn.hms.harvard.edu/flash/2016/deadly-biology-lead-exposure/.

Great Plains Laboratory. (2019). *DPP-IV: a key enzyme in food sensitivities and virtually all human physiology*. https://www.greatplainslaboratory.com/dppiv. Accessed 11 Jan 2020.

Greenblatt, J. (2018, May 24) *integrative therapies for schizophrenia and psychosis, Module 1* [Webinar]. Retrieved from: https://isom.ca/schizophrenia-psychosis/.

Hoffer, A. (2001a). Thyroid and schizophrenia. *Journal of Orthomolecular Medicine*, *16*(4), 205–212.

Hoffer, A., & Osmond, H. (1963). Malvaria: A new psychiatric disease. *Acta Psychiatrica Scandinavica*, *39*(2), 335–366. doi: 10.1111/j.1600-0447.1963.tb07470.x.

Inan-Eroglu, E., & Ayaz, A. (2018). Is aluminum exposure a risk factor for neurological disorders? Journal of Research in Medical Sciences : *The Official Journal of Isfahan University of Medical Sciences*, *23*. https://doi.org/10.4103/jrms.JRMS_921_17.

Jeppesen, R., & Benros, M. E. (2019). Autoimmune diseases and psychotic disorders. *Frontiers in Psychiatry*, *10*, 131.

Jones, C. E., Underwood, C. K., Coulson, E. J., & Taylor, P. J. (2007). Copper induced oxidation of serotonin: Analysis of products and toxicity. *Journal of Neurochemistry*, *102*(4), 1035–1043. https://doi.org/10.1111/j.1471-4159.2007.04602.x.

Joseph, J. A., Shukitt-Hale, B., Casadesus, G., & Fisher, D. (2005). Oxidative stress and inflammation in brain aging: nutritional considerations. *Neurochemical Research*, *30*(6-7), 927-935.

Kalaydjian, A. E., Eaton, W., Cascella, N., & Fasano, A. (2006). The gluten connection: the association between schizophrenia and celiac disease. *Acta Psychiatrica Scandinavica*, *113*(2), 82-90.

Karakuła-Juchnowicz, H., Dzikowski, M., Pelczarska, A., Dzikowska, I., & Juchnowicz, D. (2016). The brain-gut axis dysfunctions and hypersensitivity to food antigens in the etiopathogenesis of schizophrenia. *Psychiatria Polska*, *50*(4), 747-760.

Kelly, D. L., Demyanovich, H. K., Eaton, W. W., Cascella, N., Jackson, J., Fasano, A., & Carpenter, W. T. (2018). Anti gliadin antibodies (AGA IgG) related to peripheral inflammation in schizophrenia. *Brain, Behavior, and Immunity*, *69*, 57-59.

Kelly, D. L., Demyanovich, H. K., Rodriguez, K. M., Cihákova, D., Talor, M. V., McMahon, R. P., ... & Fasano, A. (2019). Randomized controlled trial of a gluten-free diet in patients with schizophrenia positive for antigliadin antibodies (AGA IgG): a pilot feasibility study. *Journal of Psychiatry & Neuroscience: JPN*, *44*(3), 1-9.

Kim, T. H., & Moon, S. W. (2011). Serum homocysteine and folate levels in korean schizophrenic patients. *Psychiatry Investigation*, *8*(2), 134-140.

Levinta, A., Mukovozov, I., & Tsoutsoulas, C. (2018). Use of a gluten-free diet in schizophrenia: A systematic review. *Advances in Nutrition*, *9*(6), 824-832.

Liu, T., Lu, Q.-B., Yan, L., Guo, J., Feng, F., Qiu, J., & Wang, J. (2015). Comparative study on serum levels of 10 trace elements in schizophrenia. *PLoS ONE*, *10*(7). https://doi.org/10.1371/journal.pone.0133622.

Maqsood, R., & Stone, T. W. (2016). The gut-brain axis, BDNF, NMDA and CNS disorders. *Neurochemical Research*, *41*(11), 2819-2835.

McGinnis, W. R., Audhya, T., Walsh, W. J., Jackson, J. A., McLaren-Howard, J., Lewis, A., ... Hoffer, A. (2008). Discerning the mauve factor, Part 1. *Alternative Therapies in Health and Medicine*, *14*(2), 40–50.

Metcalf, S. A., Jones, P. B., Nordstrom, T., Timonen, M., Mäki, P., Miettunen, J., ... & Veijola, J. (2017). Serum C-reactive protein in adolescence and risk of schizophrenia in adulthood: A prospective birth cohort study. *Brain, Behavior, and Immunity*, *59*, 253-259.

Modabbernia, A., Velthorst, E., Gennings, C., De Haan, L., Austin, C., Sutterland, A., ... Reichenberg, A. (2016). Early-life metal exposure and schizophrenia: A proof-of-concept study using novel tooth-matrix biomarkers. European Psychiatry: *The Journal of the Association of European Psychiatrists*, *36*, 1–6. https://doi.org/10.1016/j.eurpsy.2016.03.006.

Neal, A. P., & Guilarte, T. R. (2010). Molecular neurobiology of lead (Pb(2+)): Effects on synaptic function. *Molecular Neurobiology*, *42*(3), 151–160. https://doi.org/10.1007/s12035-010-8146-0.

Nemani, K., Ghomi, R. H., McCormick, B., & Fan, X. (2015). Schizophrenia and the gut–brain axis. *Progress in Neuro-Psychopharmacology and Biological Psychiatry*, *56*, 155-160.

Nguyen, T. T., Kosciolek, T., Eyler, L. T., Knight, R., & Jeste, D. V. (2018). Overview and systematic review of studies of microbiome in schizophrenia and bipolar disorder. *Journal of Psychiatric Research*, *99*, 50–61. doi: 10.1016/j.jpsychires.2018.01.013.

Orisakwe, O. E. (2014). The role of lead and cadmium in psychiatry. *North American Journal of Medical Sciences*, *6*(8), 370. https://doi.org/10.4103/1947-2714.139283.

Pataracchia, R. J. (2008). Orthomolecular treatment for schizophrenia: A review (Part Two). *Journal of Orthomolecular Medicine*, *23*(2), 95–105.

Pfeiffer, C. (1974). Observations on trace and toxic elements in hair and serum. *Orthomolecular Psychiatry*, *3*(4), 259–264.

Phensy, A., Duzdabanian, H. E., Brewer, S., Panjabi, A., Driskill, C., Berz, A., Peng, G., & Kroener, S. (2017). Antioxidant treatment with n-acetyl cysteine prevents the development of cognitive and social behavioral deficits that result from perinatal ketamine treatment. *Frontiers in Behavioral Neuroscience*, *11*. https://doi.org/10.3389/fnbeh.2017.00106.

Prousky, J. (2006). *The Orthomolecular treatment of schizophrenia*. Naturopathic Doctor News and Review. https://ndnr.com/neurology/the-orthomolecular-treatment-of-schizophrenia/.

Prousky, J. (2007, February/March). *The Orthomolecular treatment of schizophrenia: A primer for clinicians*. Townsend Letter for Doctors & Patients.

Pruimboom, L., & De Punder, K. (2015). The opioid effects of gluten exorphins: asymptomatic celiac disease. *Journal of Health, Population and Nutrition*, *33*(1), 24.

Radhakrishnan, R., Calvin, S., Singh, J. K., Thomas, B., & Srinivasan, K. (2013). Thyroid dysfunction in major psychiatric disorders in a hospital based sample. *The Indian Journal of Medical Research*, *138*(6), 888–893.

Rafati Rahimzadeh, M., Rafati Rahimzadeh, M., Kazemi, S., & Moghadamnia, A. (2017). Cadmium toxicity and treatment: An update. *Caspian Journal of Internal Medicine*, *8*(3), 135–145. https://doi.org/10.22088/cjim.8.3.135.

Roszkowska, A., Pawlicka, M., Mroczek, A., Bałabuszek, K., & Nieradko-Iwanicka, B. (2019). Non-celiac gluten sensitivity: A review. *Medicina*, *55*(6), 222.

Roth, J. A. (2006). Homeostatic and toxic mechanisms regulating manganese uptake, retention, and elimination. *Biological Research*, *39*(1), 45–57. https://doi.org/10.4067/s0716-97602006000100006.

Rowland, L. M., Demyanovich, H. K., Wijtenburg, S. A., Eaton, W. W., Rodriguez, K., Gaston, F., ... & Hong, L. E. (2017). Antigliadin antibodies (AGA IgG) are related to neurochemistry in schizophrenia. *Frontiers in Psychiatry*, *8*, 104.

Salim S. (2014). Oxidative stress and psychological disorders. *Current Neuropharmacology*, *12*(2), 140–147. https://doi.org/10.2174/1570159X11666131120230309.

Santos, N. C., Costa, P., Ruano, D., Macedo, A., Soares, M. J., Valente, J., … Palha, J. A. (2012). Revisiting thyroid hormones in schizophrenia. *Journal of Thyroid Research*, *2012*, 1–15. doi: 10.1155/2012/569147.

Schwarz E., Maukonen J., Hyytiäinen T., Kieseppä T., Orešič M., Sabunciyan S., … Suvisaari J. (2018). Analysis of microbiota in first episode psychosis identifies preliminary associations with symptom severity and treatment response. *Schizophrenia Research*, *192*, 398–403.

Sears M. E. (2013). Chelation: harnessing and enhancing heavy metal detoxification – a review. *The Scientific World Journal*, *2013*, 219840. https://doi.org/10.1155/2013/219840.

Shaw, W. (2010). Increased urinary excretion of a 3-(3-hydroxyphenyl)-3-hydroxypropionic acid (HPHPA), an abnormal phenylalanine metabolite of Clostridia spp. in the gastrointestinal tract, in urine samples from patients with autism and schizophrenia. *Nutritional Neuroscience*, *13*(3), 135–143. doi: 10.1179/147683010x12611460763968.

Specter, M. (2014). *Against the grain*. New Yorker Magazine.

Sturgeon, C., & Fasano, A. (2016). Zonulin, a regulator of epithelial and endothelial barrier functions, and its involvement in chronic inflammatory diseases. *Tissue Barriers*, *4*(4), e1251384.

Suboticanec, K., Folnegović-Smalc, V., Korbar, M., Mestrović, B., & Buzina, R. (1990). Vitamin C status in chronic schizophrenia. *Biological Psychiatry*, *28*(11), 959-966.

The deadly biology of lead exposure. (2016, June 27). Science in the News. http://sitn.hms.harvard.edu/flash/2016/deadly-biology-lead-exposure/.

Tomasik, J., Yolken, R. H., Bahn, S., & Dickerson, F. B. (2015). Immunomodulatory effects of probiotic supplementation in schizophrenia patients: A randomized, placebo-controlled trial. *Biomarker Insights*, *10*, 47–54. doi: 10.4137/bmi.s22007.

Tsafrir, J. (n.d.). *Copper toxicity: A common cause of psychiatric symptoms*. Psychology Today. Retrieved April 30, 2020, from https://www.psychologytoday.com/blog/holistic-psychiatry/201709/copper-toxicity-common-cause-psychiatric-symptoms.

Tye-Din, J. A., Galipeau, H., & Agardh, D. (2018). Celiac disease: a review of current concepts in pathogenesis, prevention and novel therapies. *Frontiers in Pediatrics*, *6*, 350.

US EPA, OCSPP. (2015, August 26). *How people are exposed to mercury* [Overviews and Factsheets]. US EPA. https://www.epa.gov/mercury/how-people-are-exposed-mercury.

Walsh, W., Glab, L., & Haakenson, M. (2004). Reduced violent behavior following biochemical therapy. *Physiology & Behavior*, *82*(5), 835–839. doi: 10.1016/s0031-9384(04)00310-5.

World Health Organization Regional Office for Europe Copenhagen. (2000). *Air quality guidelines for europe* (2nd ed.). WHO regional publications. http://www.euro.who.int/__data/assets/pdf_file/0005/74732/E71922.pdf.

Yang, J., Jiang, Z., Wang, Y., Qureshi, I., Phil, M., & Dong, X. (1997). Maternal-fetal transfer of metallicmercury via the placenta and milk. *Annals Of Clinical and Laboratory Science*, *27*(2). http://www.annclinlabsci.org/content/27/2/135.full.pdf.

Modulators of schizophrenia

Modulators are substances that have roles in promoting or addressing schizophrenia, depending on the amount present in the body. Modulators can have positive and negative effects.

Nutrients and health

During the golden age of vitamin discovery, between 1930 and 1940, physicians eagerly explored the use of each vitamin as it became available. The synthetic vitamins were much cheaper and could be used freely as there was little or no safety hazard.

A few pioneer physicians concentrated on a few diseases and studied them thoroughly. Drs. Wilfrid and Evan Shute in Ontario, Canada, studied the impact of vitamin E on cardiovascular disease and on burns. Dr. William Kaufman published two books describing the use of vitamin B3 for the treatment of arthritis and old age and Dr. Fred Klenner described the use of vitamin C in very large doses for a variety of very dangerous diseases including cancer.

The most important nutrient for any individual is the one that is most deficient. The best test is clinical. If a person takes a vitamin and after a while is healthier and feels better, obviously that vitamin was needed. If there is no improvement, this may be due to the dose being too little or because there are other nutrient deficiencies as well which have not been corrected.

The great biochemist Roger Williams, discoverer of folic acid and pantothenic acid, first used the orchestra analogy to explain why all the essential nutrients were needed, that one can not be more important than any other. All the musicians are equally important. The musicians play from the same score, follow the conductor and the final music depends upon each musician performing according to the way the music is written. If the pianist in a piano concerto drops out it becomes the most important one. Each instrument is essential for a harmonious production. Vitamin B3 is one of the essential components of nature's grand symphony as performed by each cell of our bodies.

Using nutrients

After first discussing the diet, patients are introduced to the vitamins and starting doses they should take. The one most frequently used is B3. Other vitamins and dosages are described along with potential side effects.

It takes about 2 months for the program to begin having positive effects. More than one vitamin or supplement may be needed and usually it is a good idea to add a multivitamin containing the full complex of B vitamins in concentration of 25-100 mg. Vitamin C is recommended as a vitamin which makes the body better able to endure stress.

Reasons for nutrient deficiencies

Modern diets seldom provide enough of the nutrients. The addition of thiamin, riboflavin and niacinamide to flour recognizes this important fact about modern foods. Therefore, it is very likely that when one nutrient is lacking, often there will be many others.

The Journal American Medical Association carried a report in which the authors recommended that every person take extra vitamins daily.

There are many possible reasons for this. Firstly, the conditions which led to the increased need for supplementation of one nutrient are also active for other nutrients.

Secondly, processed foods have lost much of their natural nutritive value. Thus white flour and white rice lacks most of its B vitamins which are present primarily in the germ and bran layers.

Thirdly, modern food is developed by plant geneticists and breeders for yield, stability and visual appeal rather than nutritive value. Modern foods are sweeter, larger, more palatable, store better and look better.

A study by Don Davis, Melvin Epp and Hugh Riordan reported that 43 crops were less rich in nutrients today compared to 50 years ago. Therefore, it makes good clinical sense to have every patient take one of the multivitamin preparations such as the B complex 50s or 100s.

Like vitamins, minerals are also lacking or greatly reduced in refined, processed foods. Soil nutrient depletion and excessive reliance on fertilizers account for much of the problem.

Nutrients and medication

Neuroleptic drugs may be needed once a disease such as schizophrenia is well established. They are used with the usual psychiatric indications and dosage.

But vitamin therapy makes medication more effective so that smaller drug doses are needed to achieve the same anti-psychotic effects. This decreases the chance of developing tardive dyskinesia and other side effects. (Tardive dyskinesia is discussed in more detail on page 62).

Patients on orthomolecular therapy start to respond to the anti-psychotics sooner and this is an indication that their dose can be decreased very slowly and cautiously, as these drugs are very addictive and have a severe withdrawal effect if they are suddenly discontinued.

The optimal drug dose is that which controls the symptoms without inducing others that are incapacitating. With the atypical anti-psychotics, attention must be given to the metabolic changes that are induced such as excessive weight gain, increased cholesterol and triglyceride levels and increased incidence of diabetes.

Niacin

There are two main forms of nicotinic acid known medically as niacin and nicotinamide. The term vitamin B3 refers to these two and to the nicotinamide adenine dinucleotide system, NAD and NADH.

NADH is the reduced form and more active than NAD. The term vitamin B3 deficiency means a deficiency of niacin, or of niacinamide or of nicotinamide adenine dinucleotide (NAD) or its reduced derivative NADH.

I have been amazed for the past 50 years about the remarkable versatility and usefulness of vitamin B3, especially niacin. I've concluded that at least half the population needs extra niacin ranging from a little more than is present in our food to the large doses that have to be used to correct blood lipid levels and treat schizophrenia.

Foster and I (Hoffer & Foster, 2005) hypothesize that humanity is in the middle of a major evolutionary change in which the body is becoming more and more dependent on the amount of vitamin which is present in food. The body has used two main sources. The first is the amino acid tryptophan. About 1.6 percent of this is converted into vitamin B3. But if there are adequate amounts of this vitamin in the food, why would the body need two sources?

Linus Pauling pointed out that there was an evolutionary advantage in dropping the enzyme that converted glucose into ascorbic acid if ample supplies were present in the food. But this became a major disadvantage when the food could no longer provide the vitamin. As a result we all suffer from a vitamin C deficiency.

If the enzymes that convert tryptophan were dropped because there is enough B3 in the food, the tryptophan no longer needed to make the vitamin would be used for other purposes such as increasing the formation of serotonin. Serotonin is a very important neurotransmitter and is present in large amounts in the gut and the brain.

Roles of vitamin B3

B3 is strongly anti-oxidant. It is needed for the NADPH which is required for reduction of glutathione. B3 is a potent free-radical quencher, protecting both lipids and proteins from oxidation. It blocks nitric-oxide associated neurotoxicity.

Normally, the body maintains relatively high vitamin B3 tissue levels, which can serve a very important anti-oxidant function. At usual physiologic concentrations, B3 exceeds the anti-oxidant effects of ascorbate in some studies.

Vitamin B3 antagonists increase lipoxidation. Low vitamin B3 decreases metallothionein and increases apoptosis in brain cells. In experimental mitochondrial toxicity, B3 is neuroprotective.

Vitamin B3 deficiency

We suggested that when mankind began to convert whole grains into the modern refined white flours, about 1800, there was a major decrease in the amount of available vitamin B3, as this vitamin is located mainly in the wheat germ and bran layers.

Following this dramatic decrease in supply, the former advantages become a major disadvantage and a major part of the population suffers from a deficiency of this important vitamin.

The deficiency that is mild will not express itself for many years. But as I have shown, a prolonged period of deficiency leads to a dependency so that much larger amounts will be needed to compensate for the many years of mild to moderate deficiency.

When humanity ensures that there are adequate amounts of this very cheap vitamin from infancy on, the advantages will be re established and the disadvantages removed. The addition of vitamins to flour mandated by the United States in 1942 is a first major step in this direction.

Vitamin B3 and apparent toxicity

Usually toxicity is discussed last not first. But I want to dispose immediately of the notion that niacin is toxic to the liver. This myth, which is pervasive in medicine, is based upon a series of observations some of which were dead wrong.

Between 1940 and 1950 when the toxicity of niacin and niacinamide was studied, the LD-50 on rats was determined (LD stands for "Lethal Dose"). The LD 50 is a test used to test toxicity and is defined as the amount of a compound that will kill one half of the population of animals. If 100 mice are given 5 g of a drug and half die, 5 g is the LD-50 for that drug.

For niacin it is very high, about 4.5 g per kilogram. This is equivalent to 225 g (nearly half a pound) for a 110 pound female and 360 g for a 176 pound male or approximately 100 times as much as is normally recommended. At autopsy the animals showed elevated fatty acids in the liver

In 1950, deficiency of methyl groups was a popular topic. It caused fatty livers. Niacin and niacinamide are methyl acceptors. It therefore made sense to consider that too much vitamin B3 would cause fatty acid livers by producing a methyl deficiency syndrome.

However Professor R. Altschul, University of Saskatchewan, could not confirm these findings. In his animal studies he found that the vitamin had no effect on the fatty acid levels in the liver.

The second observation which is still routinely made is that in some patients niacin will increase liver function tests. It is assumed, incorrectly, that elevated liver function tests always means underlying liver pathology.

Many other medicines cause the same elevations of liver function tests. Usually after a few days off niacin the test results become normal. But to prevent confusing liver damage with increased activity it is best to stop the niacin for five days and then to do the tests.

The Mayo Clinic examined the livers of a series of their patients on niacin being treated for high blood cholesterol using the electron microscope and they found no evidence of pathology. This was first reported by Dr. W. Parsons Jr. (Parsons, 1964). He points out that an increase in the liver function tests, unless they are very substantial i.e. over three fold, do not indicate liver pathology.

In most patients with elevated liver function tests, the values become normal in a few days even if the niacin is not discontinued.

We advise all doctors that they should stop the niacin for at least five days before doing the test. With real liver pathology they will not be normal in five days but when they are elevated with niacin they are normal within these five days.

There are many compounds that elevate liver enzymes including all the statin drugs and many modern drugs.

Gonzalez-Heydrich, Leichtner, & Messacappa, 2003, gave 12 children a combination of olanzapine and divalproic acid. Every child had an elevated enzyme peak and in five children it remained elevated for many months. Two children had to be removed from the study because of severe pathology, pancreatitis in one and steatohepatitis in the other.

Over 40 years ago there were a few reports of liver damage and one or two deaths. These were traced to poorly made slow-release preparations, not to standard preparations.

I have used niacin for lowering cholesterol and both forms for treating schizophrenic patients since 1953 and have treated thousands of patients. Very few patients became jaundiced.

One patient recovering from schizophrenia on niacin became jaundiced. When the niacin was stopped the jaundice cleared, his schizophrenia came back. When the niacin was resumed, his schizophrenia cleared again and the jaundice did not.

I have seen no cases of jaundice in the past 20 years. But it is possible that the liver function tests may be increased due to methyl depletion. According to Professor David Capuzzi (Cappuzi, 2002), of Philadelphia, one of the world's authorities on niacin and cholesterol, this can be prevented by giving patients 1.2 g of lecithin in the morning and again at night. Betaine may also be effective (McCarty, 2000).

A young female teenaged schizophrenic patient given a month's supply, 200 tablets of niacin, each 500 mg, became angry at her mother and the next day swallowed the whole bottle. For three days thereafter she had a sore abdomen.

Another teen schizophrenic after reading a paperback book on megavitamins and schizophrenia could not find any physician to monitor her. She began to increase the dose and when she reached 60 g niacin daily, all the voices she was hearing stopped. Two years later her maintenance dose was 3 g.

But even though it is safer than almost all the over-the-counter non-nutrient preparations, there is above all the most important safety rule. Whenever one takes anything and then notes a reaction which was not there before which is unpleasant and worrying they should immediately contact the physician who recommended or prescribed it.

There are a few side effects which may be a nuisance but are not toxic reactions (Hoffer, 1962; McCracken, 1994). Apart from a very few subjects who are allergic to the pills, either the active component or some of the fillers, most of these reactions are dose-related. Patients must be informed of the possible side effects both positive and negative.

The niacin flush (vasodilation)

Niacin usually causes a flush a few minutes after it is taken. A few people will flush with 25 mg, more with 50 and most with 100 mg.

The flush begins in the forehead and works its way down the body rarely affecting the toes. The higher the initial dose the greater is the initial flush, but if any dose causes a maximum flush a larger dose taken later will not cause any greater flush.

The capillaries are dilated and the blood flow through the organs is increased. There is an internal increase in blood in flow as well as in the skin. It may last up to several hours. Patients must be warned that this will happen. If not they may be very surprised and even shocked.

Patients can be started on lower doses until they have adjusted to the decreased intensity of the flush. Then the doses may be increased gradually.

Each time the niacin is taken, the flush is repeated but to a much lesser degree and in most cases after a week or so it is almost all gone and is a minor nuisance at worst.

However some do not tolerate the flush and they will have to discontinue the niacin. If the routine is interrupted several days and then resumed the same sequence of flushing will occur but the initial flush will usually not be as strong as the original one was. Non-flush preparations are available for these subjects.

The intensity of the flush is minimized by taking the pills after meals and by taking them regularly three times daily.

I have been taking it for fifty years and at the maximum have very minor flushes. It is a drier flush not like the wet menopausal flush or the flush suffered by male hormone blockers used in treating prostate cancer.

Niacinamide does not cause flushing except in about 1% of the subjects in whom will cause a very unpleasant flush, and for these people it cannot be used. Probably they convert the niacinamide too rapidly into niacin.

Vasodilation is sometimes very helpful. Many patients, particularly arthritics, have reported that they feel much better when their joints are warmed up by the flush and some will stop taking niacin for a few days in order to once more experience the flush. But for most, the sensation is not pleasant. It is tolerable if the patients knows what to expect and are properly prepared by the physician.

In a guide for patients, updated in 2018 by his long-time assistant Frances Fuller, Dr. Hoffer explained ways to mitigate the niacin flush. Actions to take include:

- taking 2 to 4 g of vitamin C at beginning of meal, and the niacin at the end of the meal (vitamin C decreases the flush by neutralizing histamine in the blood);
- taking the niacin with a cold beverage;
- avoiding hot showers or baths immediately after taking niacin; and
- starting with a lower amount of niacin and gradually increasing the daily dose—for example starting with 125 mg, then doubling the amount every 4–5 days (flushing should stop shortly after reaching 1,000 mg per day).

Chronic exposure to allergens, either food-based or environmental, can stimulate continuous production of histamine. This ongoing supply of histamine can be a reason why some people continue to flush, even after long-term niacin supplementation.

Positive side effects of niacin supplementation

If a patient takes niacin to normalize blood lipids and as a result of the vitamin activity feels very much better in other areas such as more energy, faster healing, etc., this is a positive side effect.

There are other positive side-effects that often occur. For example if the patient takes niacin to deal with his arthritis and at the same time his cholesterol levels decrease, this result would be a major positive side effect or better still a side benefit.

Niacin lowers C-reactive protein. This is one of the markers of inflammation. The statins also lower CRP but in contrast to the statins, niacin is not toxic.

In common with all water-soluble nutrients, niacin is compatible with all foods and with medication. It reinforces the therapeutic effect of antipsychotic medications so that the dose of these powerful drugs can be reduced.

No-flush vitamin B3

No-flush and slow-release preparations, which are also no-flush, are available. The best no-flush product is inositol hexaniacinate, which is an ester of inositol, a vitamin and niacin. I have used it for many years with success and have considered it as valuable as niacin. But I have not used it routinely as my first choice because of its cost and because so many of my patients cannot afford it and it is not covered by medical plans.

Uncommon side effects of niacin supplementation

Other uncommon side effects are increased gastric acidity probably because niacin does stimulate secretion of gastric juice, and increased brown pigmentation of certain areas of the skin, usually the flexor surfaces. This is not acanthosis nigricans, a very serious condition, even though it has been erroneously labeled as such.

This is never a problem for patients if they are told the truth but is a problem for some doctors who are not familiar with it.

Acanthosis nigricans is a very serious, almost cancer like condition. Parsons correctly called the increased skin condition a skin change which resembles acanthosis nigricans. It does this but only in color, not in pathology.

The browning effect of niacin on a very few subjects is entirely different. It is transient, usually lasting only a few months and when it is clear the skin is perfectly normal and never recurs even with continued use. I think it is due to the deposition of melanin-containing indoles from tyrosine and adrenalin. It occurs most commonly in schizophrenic patients and is part of the healing process.

Vitamin B3 and adrenochrome

Vitamin B3's prime mechanism of action in regards to schizophrenia involves its ability to decrease the production adrenochrome. (Hoffer, 1999).

Vitamin B3 accepts methyl groups which would otherwise be used to produce adrenaline. As well, vitamin B3 acts as an antioxidant to prevent the oxidation of adrenalin to adrenochrome (Prousky, 2006).

Supplementing vitamin B3

Jonathan Prousky, ND
The Orthomolecular Treatment of Schizophrenia:
A Primer for Clinicians
(Prousky, 2007)

The starting dose of niacin for adults is 1,000 mg three times daily. In my opinion, the daily dose needs to be slowly increased to 4,500-18,000 mg to achieve the best possible outcome.

At 3,000 mg daily, the flush and other symptoms will cease to be an issue following the first two to three days of treatment and will practically disappear thereafter. If patients are not consistently taking these high-milligram doses throughout the day, they will continually re-experience these cutaneous reactions.

The concern over liver toxicity is very minor if immediate-release niacin preparations are used (Mullen, Greenspan, & Mitchell, 1989; Hoffer, 1995). Sustained-release preparations (and likely other preparations such as timed- or slow-release ones) can cause liver toxicity and are not recommended for schizophrenic patients unless under close supervision (Hoffer, 1983). In my clinical experience, niacin is more effective and better tolerated than niacinamide for schizophrenia.

Some patients prefer niacinamide, since it does not cause flushing as well as the other cutaneous reactions. Nausea and dry mouth are much more common with the use of niacinamide than with niacin. The daily dosages of niacinamide should not exceed 6,000 mg, since the likelihood of nausea accompanied with vomiting is much greater (Brody, Preut, Schornmer, & Schurmeyer, 2002).

In 8 years of managing schizophrenic patients on very high therapeutic doses of niacin, I have not had a single case where the vitamin had to be discontinued due to transaminitis (high levels of transaminases liver enzymes) or hepatotoxicity.

Vitamin B6 (pyridoxine)

Vitamin B6 is strongly anti-oxidant. The active form of vitamin B6, Pyridoxal-5-phosphate (P5P), is required for synthesis of glutathione, metallothionein, CoQ10 and heme, all of which play very important anti-oxidant roles.

With zinc, P5P is required for the enzyme glutamic acid decarboxylase (GAD), needed by the body to block excitotoxicity which would otherwise increase oxidative stress.

P5P protects vulnerable enzyme lysinyl groups from oxidation, specifically in the case of glutathione peroxidase.

Vitamin B6 deficiency and oxidative stress

Even marginal B6 deficiency lowers glutathione peroxidase and glutathione reductase, promoting mitochondrial decay and raising measurable lipid peroxide levels.

Thus, there exist numerous ways by which impaired vitamin B6 function and oxidative stress reciprocate. Hydroxyl radical and superoxide even attack vitamin B6 vitamers directly. High doses of B6 may compensate oxidatively-impaired enzyme and co-enzyme function in high-mauve subjects.

Supplementing vitamin B6

The daily dose ranges of pyridoxine ranges from 100 mg to 1 g. Early in the development of orthomolecular psychiatry, the pioneer physicians freely used up to 3 g daily and did not see any complications.

But this vitamin was given a bad reputation following a survey in which the author located 6 patients in several medical schools who were taking between 2 and 6 g daily. These six suffered from neurological changes in their feet from which they recovered fully after this vitamin was stopped.

The standard medical literature incorrectly considers it one of the dangerous vitamins. The doses seldom need to be larger than 250 mg taken three times daily.

Pyridoxine may increase hyperactivity in some children. However having the child take magnesium prevents this.

Vitamin B6 supplementation improves tardive dyskinesia and parkinsonian symptoms

Fifteen patients with schizophrenia and schizoaffective disorder were given 400 mg/day of vitamin B6 for 9 weeks in addition to their antipsychotic medication. Supplementation significantly improved tardive dyskinesia and parkinsonian symptoms (Miodownik, Cohen, Kotler, & Lerner, 2003).

Vitamin C (ascorbic acid)

Vitamin C plays a major role in physical medicine, especially in the treatment of cancer. In mental illnesses it is not as relevant as are the B vitamins, but due to its anti-stress properties, it is advantageous to use 1 to 3 g daily for all patients. It is remarkably safe.

Vitamin C is required for the synthesis of many compounds important for normal mental health. Some of these are:
- tyrosine,
- thyroxine,
- norepinephrine,
- epinephrine,
- serotonin,
- carnitine, and
- corticosteroids.

The antioxidant function of vitamin C is important in the context of schizophrenia because, along with vitamin B3, it prevents the oxidation of adrenalin to adrenochrome (Smythies, 1996; Hoffer, 1999), and helps patient cope by moderating stress (Hoffer, 1977).

More vitamin C needed with schizophrenia

It was first reported in 1942 that schizophrenics receiving an adequate amount of dietary vitamin C from diet had lower blood levels of vitamin C than people in good health (Horwitt, 1942). Studies in 1960s found chronic psychiatric patients required much higher vitamin C doses in order to excrete it in normal amounts in the urine.

Vitamin C deficiency greater in schizophrenics

One hundred and six recently hospitalized schizophrenic patients were given a loading test of vitamin C.

Seventy-six percent of the patients were deficient versus 30% of the controls; 22% of the patients had significant deficiency versus 1% of controls (Pauling, 1974).

Smoking and vitamin C

Smoking depletes vitamin C in the body. People who smoke require an additional 35 mg/day of vitamin C versus nonsmokers. (Institute of Medicine 2000)

Vitamin C and medications

Vitamin C has been shown beneficial and safe, when used in conjunction with schizophrenia medications.

Adjunctive vitamin C improves symptoms

In a study by Beauclair et al., 13 schizophrenia patients who had stabilized on antipsychotics but had residual symptoms received vitamin C supplements, gradually increasing from 1 to 8 g/day.

After 8 weeks 20% of the patients showed improvement on the psychiatric rating scale, and 35% showed improvement on the Clinical Global Impressions (CGI) Scale (Beauclair, Vinogradov, Riney, Csernansky, & Hollister, 1987).

Vitamin C improves newly-diagnosed schizophrenia symptoms

Forty newly-diagnosed schizophrenics taking atypical antipsychotics were randomized to receive either vitamin C 500 mg/day or placebo for 8 weeks.

The treatment group showed significant improvement in Brief Psychiatric Rating Scale and in serum malondialdehyde (MDA) (a marker for oxidative stress) levels (Dakhale, Khanzode, Khanzode, & Saoji, 2005).

Case study: adjunctive vitamin C improves mental health

A 39 year-old male with schizoaffective disorder who was unresponsive to various medications and remained severely psychotic, was given vitamin C (2 g/day) in addition to his regimen of chlorpromazine (250 mg/day), haloperidol (50 mg/day), and carbamazepine (800 mg/day)

Improvement in mental state was seen within 2 weeks. His circumstantial and tangential thinking, delusions, and hallucinations almost completely disappeared. His Haloperidol dosing was reduced to 14 mg/day and vitamin C increased to 8 g/day without affecting his mental status. The patient reported the addition of vitamin C was instrumental in improving his symptoms enabling him to be discharged (Sandyk & Kanofsky, 1993).

Supplementing vitamin C

A common effect when large doses are used is loosening of the stools. This is not real diarrhea as there is no pain and cramps. But if it occurs, the dose should be decreased to below this level.

Jonathan Prousky, ND
The Orthomolecular Treatment of Schizophrenia: A Primer for Clinicians
Townsend Letter February/March 2007

Vitamin C is also an effective anti-stress nutrient that helps schizophrenic patients cope more effectively (Hoffer, 1977). There is recent evidence that high-dose vitamin C (3,000 mg of sustained-release daily) is indeed an anti-stress nutrient, since it was able to subjectively reduce psychological stress, decrease blood pressure, and lower cortisol levels in healthy men after 14 days of use (Meister, 1994).

A report by Smythies described additional roles that vitamin C has upon the brain including the following:

1. the ability to protect NMDA receptors from glutamate toxicity within the brain,

2. antagonism of the effects of amphetamines,

3. enhancement of older APDs like haloperidol, and

4. the ability to prevent the auto-oxidation of dopamine to its toxic derivatives (Baez, Segura-Aguilar, Widerslen, Johansson, & Mannervik, 1997).

Vitamin C also conserves intracellular glutathione and is likely a redox glutathione cofactor (Pauling et al., 1973). This is important since glutathione S-transferases are important enzymes that facilitate the conjugation of glutathione to adrenochrome, dopaminochrome, and noradrenochrome and render these toxic metabolites non-toxic (Suboticanec, Folnegović-Smalc, Korbar, M., Mestrović, & Buzina, 1990).

The gene for glutathione S-transferase is defective in schizophrenia (Smythies, 2002). I believe that this defect might be partially remedied by supplementation with high dosages of vitamin C, which would preserve glutathione in its reduced state and increase the amount of available glutathione that could be used for the synthesis of the glutathione S-transferase enzyme.

Dr. Prousky also wrote about vitamin C dosing in *Naturopathic Doctor News and Review* (Prousky, 2006):

"Vitamin C should be prescribed at 1,000 mg three times daily, and increased until the sub-laxative dose has been reached (i.e., the dose just below the one that produces diarrhea). A few clinical studies have shown both acute and chronic schizophrenic patients to require high-gram doses of this vitamin in order to saturate tissue stores (Pauling et al., 1973; Suboticanec, et al., 1990)."

"*The absence of any substantial side effects, cheaper cost, improvement in BPRS score, and the fact that plasma ascorbic acid levels are decreased in schizophrenia and increases after oral supplementation make it a particularly attractive therapeutic adjuvant in the treatment of schizophrenia.*" (Dakhale, Khanzode, Khanzode, & Saoji, 2005).

Vitamin D

Roles of vitamin D in mental health

Vitamin D, which is made from cholesterol in the skin and UVB radiation, is a neurosteroid hormone that has roles in brain development and normal brain function.

Vitamin D regulates the transcription of genes involved in pathways for synaptic plasticity, neuronal development and protection against oxidative stress (Graham et al., 2015).

Vitamin D and inflammation

Vitamin D-deficient cells produce higher levels of the inflammatory cytokines TNF-α and IL-6, while cells treated with vitamin D release significantly less.

Supplementation of vitamin D in the general population has been shown to reduce circulating amounts of CRP, demonstrating that vitamin D has anti-inflammatory properties (Chiang, Natarajan, & Fan, 2016).

Vitamin D, dopamine, and serotonin

Vitamin D has roles in dopamine and serotonin synthesis.

In the adrenal glands, vitamin D regulates tyrosine hydroxylase, which is the rate-limiting enzyme for the synthesis of dopamine, epinephrine, and norepinephrine. In the brain, vitamin D regulates the synthesis, release, and function of serotonin. Serotonin modulates executive function, sensory gating, social behaviour, and impulsivity (Patrick & Ames, 2015).

Vitamin D deficiency and brain development

Vitamin D positively influences tryptophan hydroxylase (TPH) enzymes.

Patrick & Ames (2014) found that:
- low levels of vitamin D during fetal and neonatal development impact brain development,
- low amounts of vitamin D result in lack of suppression of TPH1, which drives increased synthesis of serotonin in the gut. Increased gut serotonin promotes digestive tract inflammation, which, in turn promotes abnormal brain development, and
- low vitamin D also results in poor expression of TPH2, leading to reduced brain serotonin, which also promotes abnormal brain development.

Measuring vitamin D

The best indicator of vitamin D status is serum 25(OH)D, also known as 25-hydroxyvitamin D. 25(OH)D reflects the amount of vitamin D in the body that is produced by the skin and obtained from food and supplements.

Vitamin D levels and health status

Institute of Medicine, Food and Nutrition Board. (2010)

Serum (ng/ml)	Health status
<20	deficient
20–39	generally considered adequate
40–50	adequate <replete>
>50–60	proposed optimum health level
>200	potentially toxic

Folate (folic acid)

Folate versus folic acid

Folate is a water-soluble vitamin. "Folate" is the form that is naturally occurring in foods. Since folate is unstable, the synthetic form, "folic acid" is often used in supplements and food fortification.

Psychiatric interest in folic acid has developed over the past years.

Small amounts are added to flour in order to prevent the birth of spina bifida babies.

People with depression tend to be low in folic acid and when taken in large doses of 25 mg per day and over it has anti-depressant properties.

The fear that it will mask pernicious anemia is unjustified but pervasive and it is the reason why the 5 mg tablets are available only on prescription. Giving patients any of the current B complex preparations will provide enough B12 to assure anyone that pernicious anemia will not be covered up.

Hunter, in reviewing the need to add folic acid to flour to prevent spina bifida, wrote "Concerns about vitamin B12 originate from findings in the late 1940s that while pernicious anemia responded well to folate, the neurologic signs of B12 deficiency neither responded nor were prevented" (Hunter, 2000). Indeed, it became part of medical dogma that folate could precipitate more severe and aggressive neurologic complications.

Dickinson did a comparison of case studies and series of patients with B12 deficiency, before and after the introduction of treatment with folic acid, and found no evidence that folate increased the rate or the severity of the neurologic presentation of B12 deficiency.

About 28% of cases of B12 deficiency present neurologically, and practicing physicians should always consider this diagnosis in a patient with paresthesia, weakness, or ataxia.

Folate and mental health

Folate has important roles in maintaining mental health, including:
- the biosynthesis of neurotransmitters,
- amino acid metabolism ,
- myelination of neurons,
- DNA replication,
- regulation of gene expression,
- cell division, and
- reduction of homocysteine.

Folate deficiency

Severe folate deficiencies have been linked to increased risk of neurodevelopmental and psychiatric disorders. A 2016 meta-analysis of 20 studies including 1,463 cases showed significantly lower folate levels in schizophrenia patients (Cao et al., 2016).

MTHFR and folate

The methylenetetrahydrofolate reductase (MTHFR) enzyme converts folate to 5-MTHF (methylfolate), the most bioavailable form of folate. Methylfolate is the form of folate that crosses the blood-brain barrier.

MTHFR polymorphisms and schizophrenia

Polymorphisms in the genes that make the MTHFR enzyme result in decreased function of the enzymes and reduced conversion folate to methylfolate.

Schizophrenics are more likely to have MTHFR polymorphisms than healthy subjects. They are also more likely to have lower amounts of circulating folate and higher levels of homocysteine (El-Hadidy, Abdeen, El-Aziz, Sherin, & Al-Harrass, 2014).

Food sources of folate

Food sources of folate include:
- leafy green vegetables,
- legumes,
- avocados,
- oranges, and
- fortified grains.

Negative effects of the MTHFR polymorphism can, to a degree, be compensated for by supplementing methylated folate.

Folate reduces homocysteine and negative schizophrenia symptoms

A study by Saedisomeolia, Djalali, Moghadam, Ramezankhani, & Najmi (2011) measured serum folate and homocysteine levels in 60 schizophrenic and 60 healthy controls. Folate levels were lower and homocysteine levels were significantly higher in the schizophrenics compared to the controls.

The authors found that lower folate levels correlated with higher homocysteine levels and negative schizophrenia symptoms. As well, higher homocysteine correlated with lower cognitive function.

Folate status correlates with BDNF and PANSS scores

Song et al., (2014) tested serum folate, BDNF, homocysteine, and Positive and Negative Syndrome Scale (PANSS) scores in 46 drug-naïve, first episode schizophrenics, and thirty healthy controls.

They found serum folate levels positively correlated with BDNF levels in the schizophrenia group. Serum folate levels negatively correlated with PANSS-total and negative symptom scores, while serum homocysteine positively correlated with PANSS-total scores.

The authors concluded that low folate and BDNF levels, and elevated homocysteine levels, may have a role the development and expression of schizophrenia.

Vitamin B12

Roles of vitamin B12 in mental health

Several functions of vitamin B12 are considered important contributors to the maintenance of good mental health.

Vitamin B12 increases the production of S-adenosylmethionine (SAMe), which is required for creation of phospholipids. Phospholipids are incorporated into cell membranes and neuronal myelin sheaths. SAMe is involved in the production of monoamine neurotransmitters.

By decreasing plasma and brain homocysteine, vitamin B12 can help reduce, reverse, and normalize damaged neurons.

Other roles of vitamin B12 that support brain function include reducing inflammation, normalizing of deficient methylation processes, and correcting altered gene expression (Prousky, 2010).

Vitamin B12 deficiency

Deficiencies of vitamin B12 are often a result of poor absorption. Promoters of poor absorption include:
- low stomach acid,
- low intrinsic factor,
- celiac or Crohn's Disease,
- vegetarian or vegan diet,
- alcohol, and
- antacids.

Vitamin B12 ignored when within normal lab range

Jonathan Prousky, ND
Understanding the Serum Vitamin B12 Level and its Implications for Treating Neuropsychiatric Conditions: An Orthomolecular Perspective (Prousky, 2010)

Most clinicians do not consider vitamin B12 important unless the serum level is deficient when indicated by laboratory reference ranges.

The conclusion of the Newbold study (Newbold, 1989) was that vitamin B12 dependency disorders are common and neglected by the medical profession because:

1. the body level of vitamin B12 needed for full biological efficiency is unknown,
2. patients might have a deficiency in transporting vitamin B12 into their tissues (low levels of transcobalamin II), and
3. a large increase in a vitamin level might be needed to "force" one or more abnormal chemical reactions to proceed normally.

My clinical experience and the above-noted reports suggest the following:
- first, serum levels of vitamin B12 that are not "classically" deficient by current laboratory standards, are associated with neuropsychiatric signs and symptoms not limited to declines in cognitive functioning (i.e., neurological deficits), tiredness, affective disorders, psychosis, insomnia/sleep-wake disturbances, and even brain volume loss; and
- second, a variety of neuropsychiatric signs and symptoms improve when serum vitamin B12 levels are optimized or markedly increased following vitamin B12 treatment.

In addition to hypothesis-driven physical examination, all patients presenting with neuropsychiatric signs and symptoms should have their fasting serum vitamin B12 levels tested.

Supplementing vitamin B12

Prior research does support a clinical trial of vitamin B12 in patients with neuropsychiatric signs and symptoms (Delva, 1997).

Hydroxocobalamin and methylcobalamin are the forms of vitamin B12 that I administer for therapeutic purposes. I tend to rely exclusively on methylcobalamin when a patient presents with neurologic abnormalities, and use a combination of methyl and hydroxo forms when neurologic and psychiatric abnormalities are present.

While there is proof that an oral dose of cyanocobalamin (1,000 mcg daily for 3 years) can effectively treat patients with pernicious anemia (Berlin et al., 1978), my clinical experience has shown it to be inferior to the other forms of vitamin B12.

When treating such a diverse array of neuropsychiatric presentations, vitamin B12 (cobalamin) ranks among the most useful, versatile, safe, and effective orthomolecules at my disposal.

Vitamin B12 deficiency-induced schizophrenic symptoms

In a report by Kuo (2009), a 31-year-old Taiwanese male, who was a long-time vegetarian with minimal dairy intake, who was experiencing hallucinations and delusions. He was given a short round of antipsychotics and 1,000 μg/day methylcobalamin.

With supplementation, his serum vitamin B12 increased from 136 pg/mL to 250 pg/mL and within two weeks, his confusion abated and he had no recurring symptoms at one year follow-up.

Vitamin B12 deficiency affects homocysteine and schizophrenia symptoms

Thirty-three drug-free schizophrenia patients and thirty-five healthy controls were tested by Bouaziz et al. (2010) for folate, vitamin B12, homocysteine, and the MTHFR polymorphism.

Homocysteine was found to be higher, and vitamin B12 lower in the plasma of schizophrenia patients. As well, it was found that "homocysteine was significantly correlated to the "anhedonia-asociality" subscales of the Scale for the Assessment of Negative Symptoms".

The study concluded that schizophrenia may be linked to a B12 deficiency due to lack of dietary animal protein.

Lithium

Lithium is recognized as a nutritionally essential trace element. Lithium helps increase brain-derived neurotropic factor (BDNF) synthesis in neurons.

BDNF is a growth factor that supports differentiation, maturation and survival of neurons, and is involved in neuronal plasticity, modulation of neurotransmitters, and apoptosis.

BDNF levels are decreased by HPA axis activation and inflammatory cytokines, and are increased by probiotics, zinc, and lithium. Deficiencies of neurotropins like BDNF may be directly related to schizophrenia symptoms (Gören, 2016).

Lithium increases brain levels of neuroprotective BDNF

Cultures of cortical and hippocampal neurons were treated with sub-therapeutic and therapeutic doses of lithium by De-Paula, Gattaz, & Forlenza (2016).

They found that lithium upregulated BDNF synthesis and secretion in the neurons as well as an increase in intracellular and extracellular BDNF.

Lithium regulates genetic expression of brain-protective BDNF

Dwivedi & Zhang (2015) found that application of concentrated lithium to cultured neurons in vitro, increased BDNF-driven expression of anti-apoptotic proteins and decreased expression of pro-apoptotic proteins.

Magnesium

Several roles of magnesium are relevant to schizophrenia.

Magnesium decreases activation of the NMDA receptor which in turn, decreases excitatory neurotransmission (Bartlik, Bijlani, & Music, 2014).

The function metabotropic glutamate receptors (mGluRs) requires magnesium. These receptors regulate neuronal secretion, release, and activity of glutamate, as well as the activity of the GABA system (Boyle, Lawton, & Dye, 2017).

Enzyme systems that use the vitamins thiamine and pyridoxine (vitamin B6) require magnesium. Thiamine and pyridoxine are cofactors for enzymes that make serotonin, GABA, and melatonin (Kanofsky, & Sandyk, 1991).

Also, magnesium inhibits acetylcholine release. High acetylcholine and low serotonin are associated with negative schizophrenia symptoms (Kanofsky, & Sandyk, 1991).

Magnesium and schizophrenia

Lower levels of magnesium have been found in schizophrenia patients versus controls (Bartlik et al., 2014). Psychiatric symptoms reported with magnesium deficiency include depression, agitation, disorientation, auditory and visual hallucinations (Kanofsky, & Sandyk, 1991).

Magnesium deficiency

Causes of magnesium deficiency include:
- loss of soil magnesium due to farming practices,
- loss due to processing of food, water treatment processes (Bartlik et al., 2014),
- following the standard American diet pattern; which is high in processed and nutrient deficient foods,
- decreased magnesium levels in foods, especially cereal grains (Guo, Nazim, Liang, & Yang, 2016),
- digestive tract issues that decrease magnesium absorption (Kanofsky, & Sandyk, 1991),
- stress, which causes magnesium to be lost through urine (Deans, 2011), and
- chronically elevated cortisol, which depletes magnesium (Cuciureanu, & Vink, 2011).

Supplementing magnesium

An effective strategy for dosing magnesium is to gradually increase the amount to bowel tolerance, then reduce slightly.

Magnesium is best taken in divided doses throughout the day. Caution is required for high doses of magnesium with existing kidney disease.

Dr. Greenblatt recommended doses of 125 to 300 mg of magnesium glycinate 4 times a day for mood benefits, and 200 to 300 mg of magnesium glycinate or citrate to support sleep (Greenblatt, 2016).

Zinc

Roles of zinc

Zinc is a powerful anti-oxidant, shielding sulfhydryl groups and protecting lipids from peroxidation.

Zinc induces metallothionein, a very important anti-oxidant protein, and is a constituent of superoxide dismutase. Levels of vitamin A are maintained by sufficient zinc.

Zinc deficiency results in lower glutathione, vitamin E, glutathione sulfotransferase (GST), glutathione peroxidase and superoxide dismutase levels. In zinc deficiency, reactive oxygen species and lipid peroxides increase in tissue, membranes and mitochondria.

Zinc has anti-anxiety, antidepressant and antipsychotic effects, and is critical for regulating glutamate and NMDA receptor activity. As well, impaired release of zinc in the hippocampus is associated with psychotic symptoms (Andrews, 1990; Joshi, Akhtar, Najmi, Khuroo, & Goswami, 2012).

Gestational zinc deficiency and schizophrenia

In 1990, Andrews reported:
- fetal or perinatal zinc deficiency increases risk of developing schizophrenia later in life,
- first trimester zinc deficiency has immune effects on fetal brain development,
- evidence exists of damage to zinc-rich brain regions with zinc deficiency, and
- zinc supplementation during pregnancy may prevent psychosis in offspring

Essential fatty acids (EFAs)

After several generations of refined foods and omega-3 deprivation, depression, suicide, violence, and formerly rare and mysterious disorders, such as autism, are becoming increasingly common.

But some scientists see a correlation between the rising incidence of mental illness in the 20th century and the move away from a balanced ratio of omega-6 to omega-3 fatty acids.

Fatty acids and the brain

Fatty acids are required for neurotransmitter synthesis, release, binding, re-uptake, and degradation.

Approximately sixty percent of the dry weight of the brain is fat, and around 30 percent of fatty acids must be obtained through diet because they cannot be made by the body.

Low levels of the fatty acids eicosapentaenoic Acid (EPA) and docosahexaenoic acid (DHA) are associated with brain alterations that result in motor and visual impairments, attention and behaviour problems, and psychiatric disorders (Greenblatt, 2018).

EFAs and mental health

More than 20 placebo-controlled trials with high-dose EPA/DHA demonstrate improvements for multiple psychiatric illnesses. The strongest support is for the use of EFAs adjunctively with conventional treatments. EFA treatments appear to be most effective in the early stage of disease (Akter et al., 2011).

Supplementing EFAs

The use of EFAs was proposed by Dr. Donald Rudin and amplified by Dr. David Horrobin.

It is corroborated at several research institutes that these essential fatty acids are therapeutic for a large proportion of psychiatric conditions including schizophrenia and mood disorders. A number of preparations are available ranging from flax seed oil to the fish oils, which can be used to correct the imbalanced ratio of omega-6 to omega-3 fatty acids. Patients typically need 1 to 3 g taken three times daily.

Prousky (2007) documented the effects of EPA supplementation. "Eicosapentaenoic acid (EPA), an omega-3 fatty acid from fish, has been shown to help with both the positive (e.g., hallucinations and delusions) and negative symptoms (e.g., flat affect, depression and isolation) of schizophrenia (Emsley, Oosthuizen, & van Rensburg, 2003). The optimal therapeutic daily dose should provide at least 2 g of EPA".

Adjunctive EPA supplementation with FEP

Berger et al., (2007) randomized 80 patients aged 15-29 with FEP taking atypical antipsychotics to 2 g ethyl-EPA or placebo daily for 12 weeks.

Analysis showed that EPA-treated patients needed 20% less antipsychotic medication between weeks 4 through 6. They also had less extrapyramidal symptoms, less constipation, and fewer sexual side effects.

Amino acids

Glycine

Glycine is an inhibitory neurotransmitter that prevents excessive neuronal firing, and It serves as the main mechanism for neural deactivation.

Glycine is also a coagonist of NMDA and promotes regular functioning of the NMDA receptor. Underfunctioning of the NMDA receptor has been identified as a key contributing factor for schizophrenia.

Adjunctive glycine improves schizophrenia scores

In a study by Greenwood et al., (2018), 22 patients with schizophrenia or schizoaffective disorder on stable antipsychotic medications were given 0.6 g/kg/day of glycine for 6 weeks; 21 controls received a placebo.

The glycine supplementation, compared to the placebo, increased mismatch negativity duration, improved PANSS-Total, PANSS-Negative and PANSS-General symptoms.

Taurine

Taurine has antioxidant and anti-inflammatory properties. It scavenges oxidants, increases the production of antioxidants, reduces inflammatory cytokine production and "turns on" genes that reduce inflammation (Marcinkiewicz, & Kontny, 2014).

As well, taurine activates GABA and glycine channels, and inhibits NMDA glutamate receptors. It promotes neurogenesis and activates neural precursor/stem cells (O'Donnell et al., 2016).

Taurine and schizophrenia

Low levels of taurine have been found in the CSF of drug-naïve schizophrenia patients (O'Donnell et al., 2016).

Shirayama et al., (2010) found that higher levels of taurine in the prefrontal cortex of schizophrenics was associated with better cognitive functioning, specifically with faster information processing speed.

Taurine improves schizophrenia symptoms in first episode psychosis (FEP)

In a study by O'Donnell et al., (2016), 47 young adults with FEP on low-dose antipsychotics and treated with 4 g/day taurine for 12 weeks, saw significant improvements in symptoms as measured by the Brief Psychiatric Rating Scale (BPRS). Improvements were observed in positive and general symptoms, general function, and depressive symptoms.

The study authors concluded that adjunctive taurine is a safe and tolerable treatment for schizophrenia symptoms in FEP.

Theanine

Theanine crosses the blood-brain barrier where it increases serotonin and dopamine production, helps with GABA production, and protects against glutamate toxicity. It protects cells from damage from oxidative stress by maintaining cellular glutathione levels (L-theanine. Monograph, 2005), and promotes relaxation by stimulating alpha waves.

Theanine and schizophrenia

Adjunctive theanine supplementation and schizophrenia symptoms

In a study by Ritsner et al., (2011) 60 patients with schizophrenia or schizoaffective disorder, who were taking antipsychotics, were randomized to 400 mg/day of L-theanine or placebo for 8 weeks.

Compared to the placebo group, the patients who took L-theanine had improved anxiety, positive, and general psychopathology symptoms.

In another study, 17 patients with schizophrenia and 22 controls were studied by Ota et al. (2015). 250 mg/day of L-theanine was added to ongoing antipsychotic treatment for 8 weeks. Changes in the brain were evaluated using 1H magnetic resonance spectroscopy. The L-theanine patients had improved positive symptoms and sleep quality, as well as stabilized glutamatergic concentration in the brain.

N-acetylcysteine (NAC)

NAC is a derivative of the amino acid l-cysteine. It has roles in inflammation regulation and antioxidant production, and is required for the production of glutathione.

NAC modulates neurotransmitters including glutamate and dopamine, supports mitochondrial energy production, and provides neurotrophic support (Dean, Giorlando, & Berk, 2011).

Potential Mechanisms of Action of NAC

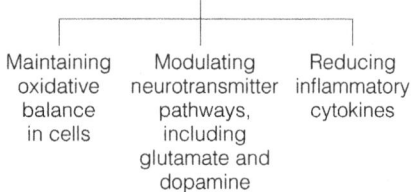

Maintaining oxidative balance in cells | Modulating neurotransmitter pathways, including glutamate and dopamine | Reducing inflammatory cytokines

(Dean, Giorlando, & Berk, 2011)

NAC and glutathione

Glutathione levels have been found to be decreased in the brains of those with schizophrenia. Although oral glutathione supplementation has poor bioavailablity, NAC supplementation has been shown to successfully raise plasma glutathione levels in those with schizophrenia (Arroll, Wilder, & Neil, 2014).

NAC impact greater with chronic schizophrenia

One hundred and twenty-one schizophrenia patients with a 12-year average illness duration were treated with 2 g/day of NAC for 24 weeks in a study by Rapado-Castro et al. (2015).

The greatest impact was in chronic schizophrenia patients (greater than 20 years duration), likely because their increased neural degeneration provided more substrate for the NAC to act upon.

The NAC supplementation was particularly beneficial for positive symptoms.

NAC is discussed in greater detail on page 71.

Medications

Ideally the aim of treatment is to restore health to its previous level or to a better level. Drugs commonly used in psychiatry do play a therapeutic role and initially, it is safer for the patients and society to bear with these toxic reactions.

Whether a drug will be used thus depends upon the relationship between its therapeutic effect and its toxic effect. Neither toxicity or efficacy can be considered alone.

A toxic drug like insulin is used safely because its therapeutic value is so great. Ideally, we want compounds that are therapeutic and non-toxic at the effective dose range. Therefore in considering whether or not to use any therapeutic substance, all these factors are taken into account and usually long usage will lay down guidelines for these compounds.

Physicians who debate the merits of therapeutic substances tend to be biased according to the paradigm they follow.

Doctors using drugs are biased in their favor and will tend to exaggerate their value and play down their side effects. Doctors who depend much more on nutrients are also biased in their favor and more likely to exaggerate their value and to minimize their possible side effects. I have no problem with this as long as the reader knows and understands the bias.

Jonathan Prousky, ND
The Orthomolecular Treatment of Schizophrenia:
A Primer for Clinicians
(Prousky, 2007)

Standard treatments use powerful atypical psychotic drugs (APDs) such as aripiprazole, clozapine, olanzapine. quetiapine, and risperidone. These drugs primarily act on dopamine receptors within the central nervous system and reduce symptoms of the disease by about 15-20%."

Additional medications are often prescribed to control the parkinsonian/extrapyramidal symptoms (e.g., involuntary movements, tremors, and rigidity) that can result from their use.

However, recent research has demonstrated that, at high dosages, the atypical APDs pose the same risks for the development of parkinsonian symptoms as do the older APDs." The majority of schizophrenic patients are also provided with a supplementary cocktail of medications consisting of benzodiazepines, antidepressants, and, sometimes, additional atypical APDs.

Schizophrenic patients taking one or two of the atypical APDs are at high risk for brain damage, cardiac arrhythmias, diabetes mellitus, sedation, sexual dysfunction, akathisia, and weight gain. Often patients experience a vague dysphoria from their medications, a sense of unease that something isn't quite right. (Horrobin, 2001)

Prousky (2006) stated that "Very few psychiatrists would consider more than 10% of his or her current schizophrenic pool of medicated patients to be recovered".

Tranquilizer psychosis

Drugs are advantageous as they work very rapidly and help bring abnormal behavior under control in a matter of days. Nutrients have the disadvantage that they work very slowly but they have the major advantage that they are non-toxic.

However, often, the drug dosages required to control schizophrenic hallucinations and delusions are very high, but this itself causes a problem.

The "tranquilizer psychosis" is a term used to describe the mental effects—lethargy, loss of interest, difficulty in concentration, loss of libido, tardive dyskinesia—which the drugs themselves exert on the patient.

The typical tranquilized patients cannot work, concentrate, or be creative. They sleep too much and lack self-confidence.

"I cannot recall a single schizophrenic patient who did not display some evidence of this tranquilized state during my initial consultation. Some features of this tranquilized state include apathy, diminished libido, difficulty reading, disorganized thoughts, fatigue and lack of concentration" (Prousky 2006).

No improvement without reducing medications

Psychiatrists must be aware that they may not see any major improvement using orthomolecular therapy until the drugs are decreased because the nutrients themselves will not reverse the tranquilizer psychosis.

Every therapeutic trial must take into account that only the optimum dose of drugs must be used, and this means that they must be gradually withdrawn as the recovery of the patient permits.

Fewer than ten percent of patients treated with drugs alone can work at the same level as before they became ill.

The dose of the drug must be evaluated every time the patient is seen. They should be seen frequently enough so that the maintenance dose does not remain too high.

By combining both nutrients and drugs one can take advantage of both therapies and minimize the disadvantages. The patients started on both will respond much more quickly. As soon as the improvement is well established the medication can be withdrawn and the nutrients allowed to maintain control.

Orthomolecular support is required

Prousky (2006) wrote about the need for orthomolecular support:

"Schizophrenic patients will remain ill and less capable of engaging in a normal quality of life as long as their treatments involve only standard medical treatments".

"Schizophrenic patients require orthomolecular support to reduce their medication need, reduce side effects and increase their chances at fully recovering. An orthomolecular substance refers to compounds found naturally in the human body, which includes amino acids, essential fatty acids, minerals and vitamins."

Tardive dyskinesia

In the early 1950s, chlorpromazine was introduced in France by Dr. H. Laborit, a surgeon, and quickly spread into psychiatry in France and later to the rest of the world. It was much less dangerous for patients than the barbiturates, acted for a longer period of time and had a remarkable tranquilizing effect. It did not calm all the patients, but it certainly made them more docile outwardly. It also had side effects as do all in this class of drugs described in the compendiums. One of the major side effects is tardive dyskinesia. In the flush of enthusiasm for these powerful drugs in the years 1955 to 1969, their side effects were ignored.

The first psychiatrist who published his observation that they caused tardive dyskinesia was given a very rough time, but this side effect was so common it could not be ignored.

Tardive dyskinesia, consisting of erratic or repetitive muscular movements, does not occur in schizophrenic patients treated by orthomolecular methods. This is probably due to the lower effective drug doses and to the independent effects of niacin itself.

Dr. Richard Kunin, one of our orthomolecular pioneers, discovered that tardive dyskinesia can be prevented by the addition of small amounts of manganese as well as niacin.

Tardive dyskinesia comes on a few months or years after starting drugs and once it develops, it is generally believed that it cannot be treated. With the addition of orthomolecular treatment and decreasing the dose of drugs, preferably to zero, it is possible get rid of the tardive dyskinesia.

Drug patents have a limited life span and if companies are to remain financially successful they must constantly develop new ones, and a major reason given for producing new drugs is "to eliminate tardive dyskinesia." They could have achieved the same goal by using orthomolecular psychiatric treatment but that would not benefit their bottom line.

The modern atypical anti-psychotics are supposed to produce less tardive dyskinesia. But they still do to a lesser degree.

But this advantage has been negated by even more serious toxic reactions such as obesity, diabetes mellitus, increased cholesterol and triglyceride levels and cardiovascular disease.

The newer drugs, according to the best modern comparison studies of them against the older drugs, are no more efficacious, have many new side effects, are addictive and, of course, are much more expensive.

By addiction I mean that it is very difficult to discontinue these compounds.

Medication withdrawal

I have been using antipsychotics ever since chlorpromazine was introduced into North America in 1955. If a patient suddenly stopped taking the medication, there was no withdrawal. They did not develop severe withdrawal symptoms the next day. On the contrary they felt better because they were liberated from the toxic side effects. However if they still needed the therapeutic effect this would become apparent weeks or months after they had stopped taking the medication.

With the atypicals I seldom have seen this. If the drug is stopped, the next day there is a sudden resurgence of symptoms.

This rapid resurgence of symptoms is similar to the effect of heroin addiction. When the heroin is stopped, the individual is in serious trouble the next day.

The new drugs are lightly bound to the receptors in the brain and one day after stopping these drugs, the receptors are liberated. This means that one must be very careful in discontinuing these modern compounds.

With Olanzapine it is not difficult to decrease the dose from 15 to 10 mg but as the dose becomes lower, the doses must be decreased more slowly. The same holds true with Risperdone. Decreasing from 10 to 5 mg daily is not difficult, but from 5 to 1 mg may take a long time.

Orthomolecular approach to medications

The objective of orthomolecular treatment is to get patients well and this means reducing the amount of medication to zero or to such a low dose that there are no side effects. This process was significantly easier with the older drugs.

There is a solution and that is to only use these anti-psychotics if they do not cause serious, toxic side effects. If there is no alternative, then one must prescribe as small a dose as possible.

Improving diet and adding optimum amounts of the correct vitamins will not cause tardive dyskinesia or any of the serious modern toxic side effects. On the contrary orthomolecular treatment will treat and prevent them.

References

Akter, K., Gallo, D. A., Martin, S. A., Myronyuk, N., Roberts, R. T., Stercula, K., & Raffa, R. B. (2011). A review of the possible role of the essential fatty acids and fish oils in the aetiology, prevention or pharmacotherapy of schizophrenia. *Journal of Clinical Pharmacy and Therapeutics*, *37*(2), 132–139. doi: 10.1111/j.1365-2710.2011.01265.x.

Andrews, R. R. (1990). Unification of the findings in schizophrenia by reference to the effects of gestational zinc deficiency. *Medical Hypotheses*, *31*(2), 141-153.

Arroll, M. A., Wilder, L., & Neil, J. (2014). Nutritional interventions for the adjunctive treatment of schizophrenia: a brief review. *Nutrition Journal*, *13*(1), 91.

Baez, S., Segura-Aguilar, J., Widersten, M., Johansson, A. S., & Mannervik, B. (1997). Glutathione transferases catalyse the detoxication of oxidized metabolites (o-quinones) of catecholamines and may serve as an antioxidant system preventing degenerative cellular processes. *Biochemical Journal*, *324*(Pt 1), 25–28.

Bartlik, B., Bijlani, V., & Music, D. (2014, July 22). Magnesium: An essential supplement for psychiatric patients—Psychiatry Advisor. *Psychiatry Advisor*. https://www.psychiatryadvisor.com/home/therapies/magnesium-an-essential-supplement-for-psychiatric-patients/

Beauclair, L., Vinogradov, S., Riney, S. J., Csernansky, J. G., & Hollister, L. E. (1987). An adjunctive role for ascorbic acid in the treatment of schizophrenia?. *Journal Of Clinical Psychopharmacology*, *7*(4), 282-283.

Berger, G. E., Proffitt, T.-M., McConchie, M., Yuen, H., Wood, S. J., Amminger, G. P., … McGorry, P. D. (2007). Ethyl-eicosapentaenoic acid in first-episode psychosis: A randomized, placebo-controlled trial. *The Journal of Clinical Psychiatry*, *68*(12), 1867–1875. https://doi.org/10.4088/jcp.v68n1206

Berlin, R., Berlin, H., Brante, G., & Pilbrant, Å. (2009). Vitamin b12 body stores during oral and parenteral treatment of pernicious anaemia. *Acta Medica Scandinavica*, *204*(1-6), 81–84. doi: 10.1111/j.0954-6820.1978.tb08402.x.

Bouaziz, N., Ayedi, I., Sidhom, O., Kallel, A., Rafra, R., Jomaa, R., & ... El Hechmi, Z. (2010). Plasma homocysteine in schizophrenia: Determinants and clinical correlations in Tunisian patients free from antipsychotics. *Psychiatry Research*, *179*(1), 24-29.

Boyle, N. B., Lawton, C., & Dye, L. (2017). The effects of magnesium supplementation on subjective anxiety and stress—A Systematic review. *Nutrients*, *9*(5). https://doi.org/10.3390/nu9050429

Brody, S., Preut, R., Schommer, K., & Schürmeyer, T. H. (2002). A randomized controlled trial of high dose ascorbic acid for reduction of blood pressure, cortisol, and subjective responses to psychological stress. *Psychopharmacology*, *159*(3), 319–324. https://doi.org/10.1007/s00213-001-0929-6.

Cao, B., Wang, D. F., Xu, M. Y., Liu, Y. Q., Yan, L. L., Wang, J. Y., & Lu, Q. B. (2016). Lower folate levels in schizophrenia: a meta-analysis. *Psychiatry Research*, *245*, 1-7.

Cappuzi D. (2002) Personal communication.

Chiang, M., Natarajan, R., & Fan, X. (2016). Vitamin D in schizophrenia: a clinical review. *Evidence-based Mental Health*, *19*(1), 6.

Cuciureanu, M. D., & Vink, R. (2011). *Magnesium and stress*. In R. Vink & M. Nechifor (Eds.), Magnesium in the Central Nervous System. University of Adelaide Press. http://www.ncbi.nlm.nih.gov/books/NBK507250/

Dakhale, G. N., Khanzode, S. D., Khanzode, S. S., & Saoji, A. (2005). Supplementation of vitamin C with atypical antipsychotics reduces oxidative stress and improves the outcome of schizophrenia. *Psychopharmacology*, *182*(4), 494-498.

De-Paula, V. J., Gattaz, W. F., & Forlenza, O. V. (2016). Long-term lithium treatment increases intracellular and extracellular brain-derived neurotrophic factor (BDNF) in cortical and hippocampal neurons at subtherapeutic concentrations. *Bipolar Disorders*, *18*(8), 692-695.

Dean, O., Giorlando, F., & Berk, M. (2011). N-acetylcysteine in psychiatry: current therapeutic evidence and potential mechanisms of action. *Journal of Psychiatry and Neuroscience*, *36*(2), 78-86.

Deans, E. (2011, June 12). *Magnesium and the brain: The original chill pill*. Psychology Today. http://www.psychologytoday.com/blog/evolutionary-psychiatry/201106/magnesium-and-the-brain-the-original-chill-pill

Delva, M. D. (1997). Vitamin B12 replacement. To B12 or not to B12? *Canadian Family Physician*, *43*, 917–922.

Dwivedi, T., & Zhang, H. (2015). Lithium-induced neuroprotection is associated with epigenetic modication of specific BDNF gene promoter and altered expression of apoptotic-regulatory proteins. *Frontiers In Neuroscience*, *8*, 457.

El-Hadidy, M. A., Abdeen, H. M., El-Aziz, A., Sherin, M., & Al-Harrass, M. (2014). MTHFR gene polymorphism and age of onset of schizophrenia and bipolar disorder. *BioMed Research International*, *2014*, 318483.

Emsley, R., Oosthuizen, P., & van Rensburg, S. J. (2003). Clinical potential of omega-3 fatty acids in the treatment of schizophrenia. *CNS Drugs*, *17*(15), 1081-1091.

Gören, J. L. (2016). Brain-derived neurotrophic factor and schizophrenia. *Mental Health Clinician*, *6*(6), 285–288. https://doi.org/10.9740/mhc.2016.11.285.

Graham, K. A., Keefe, R. S., Lieberman, J. A., Calikoglu, A. S., Lansing, K. M., & Perkins, D. O. (2015). Relationship of low vitamin D status with positive, negative and cognitive symptom domains in people with rst-episode schizophrenia. *Early Intervention in Psychiatry*, *9*(5), 397-405.

Greenblatt, J. (2016, November 17). *Magnesium: The Missing Link in Mental Health?* The Great Plains Laboratory, Inc. Retrieved May 25, 2020, from https://www.greatplainslaboratory.com/articles-1/2016/11/17/magnesium-the-missing-link-in-mental-health

Greenblatt, J. (2018, May 24) *Integrative therapies for schizophrenia and psychosis, Module 1* [Webinar]. Retrieved from: https://isom.ca/schizophrenia-psychosis/.

Greenwood, L., Leung, S., Michie, P. T., Green, A., Nathan, P. J., Fitzgerald, P., & ... Croft, R. J. (2018). The effects of glycine on auditory mismatch negativity in schizophrenia. *Schizophrenia Research, 191*, 61-69.

Guo, W., Nazim, H., Liang, Z., & Yang, D. (2016). Magnesium deficiency in plants: An urgent problem. *The Crop Journal, 4*(2), 83–91. https://doi.org/10.1016/j.cj.2015.11.003

Hoffer A. (1999). The adrenochrome hypothesis and psychiatry. *Journal of Orthomolecular Medicine, 14*, 49-62.

Hoffer, A. (1962). *Niacin therapy in psychiatry.* CC Thomas. Springfield Ill.

Hoffer, A. (1977). *Treatment of schizophrenia.* In R. Williams, D. Kalita (Eds.), A Physician's Handbook on Orthomolecular Medicine. Keats Publishing.

Hoffer, A. (1983). Oxidation reduction and the brain. *Journal of Orthomolecular Psychiatry, 12*, 292–301.

Hoffer, A. (1998). *Vitamin B-3 & schizophrenia*. Discovery, Recovery, Controversy (pp. 28–76). Quarry Press.

Hoffer, A. (1999). The adrenochrome hypothesis and psychiatry. *Journal of Orthomolecular Medicine, 14*, 49-62.

Hoffer, A. (2001b). *Vitamin B-3 and schizophrenia.* Townsend Letter for Doctors & Patients, 213, 20–23.

Hoffer, A. (2004). Atypical anti-psychotics create dependency disorders. *Journal of Orthomolecular Medicine, 19*, 3–10.

Hoffer, A. and Foster, H. *Niacin deficiency pandemic.* In preparation 2005.

Horrobin, D. (2001). *Madness of Adam and Eve* (pp. 149–151). London, England: Corgi Books.

Horwitt, M.K. (1942). Ascorbic acid requirements of individuals in a large institution. *Proceedings of the Society for Experimental Biology and Medicine, 49*, 248-250.

Hunter, A. (2000). Fortification of foods with folic acid and vitamin B12: Definitive Action is Overdue. *Annals of the Royal College of Physicians and Surgeons Canada, 33*, 172-175.

Institute of Medicine, Food and Nutrition Board. (2010). *Dietary reference intakes for calcium and vitamin D.* Washington, DC: National Academy Press.

Joshi, M., Akhtar, M., Najmi, A. K., Khuroo, A. H., & Goswami, D. (2012). Effect of zinc in animal models of anxiety, depression and psychosis. *Human & Experimental Toxicology, 31*(12), 1237-1243.

Kanofsky, J. D., & Sandyk, R. (1991). Magnesium deficiency in chronic schizophrenia. *International Journal of Neuroscience, 61*(1–2), 87–90. https://doi.org/10.3109/00207459108986275

Kuo, S. C., Yeh, C. B., Yeh, Y. W., & Tzeng, N. S. (2009). Schizophrenia-like psychotic episode precipitated by cobalamin deficiency. *General Hospital Psychiatry, 31*(6), 586-588.

L-theanine. Monograph. (2005). *Alternative Medicine Review: A Journal of Clinical Therapeutic, 10*(2), 136–138.

Marcinkiewicz, J., & Kontny, E. (2014). Taurine and inflammatory diseases. *Amino Acids, 46*(1), 7-20.

McCarty, M., (2000). Co-administration of equimolar doses of betaine may alleviate the hepatotoxic risk associated with niacin therapy. *Medical Hypotheses, 55*, 189-194.

McCracken R. (1994). *Niacin and human health disorders.* Hygea Publishing Co, Fort Collins, Colorado.

Meister, A. (1994). Glutathione, ascorbate, and cellular protection. *Cancer Research, 54*(7 Supplement), 1969s–1975s.

Miodownik, C., Cohen, H., Kotler, M., & Lerner, V. (2003). Vitamin B6 add-on therapy in treatment of schizophrenic patients with psychotic symptoms and movement disorders. *Harefuah, 142*(8-9), 592-6.

Mullin, G. E., Greenson, J. K., & Mitchell, M. C. (1989). Fulminant hepatic failure after ingestion of sustained-release nicotinic acid. *Annals of Internal Medicine, 111*(3), 253–255. https://doi.org/10.7326/0003-4819-111-3-253.

Newbold, H. L. (1989). Vitamin B-12: Placebo or neglected therapeutic tool? *Medical Hypotheses, 28*(3), 155–164. https://doi.org/10.1016/0306-9877(89)90044-3.

O'Donnell, C. P., Allott, K. A., Murphy, B. P., Yuen, H. P., Proffitt, T. M., Papas, A., ... & Simpson, R. (2016). Adjunctive taurine in first-episode psychosis: A phase 2, double-blind, randomized, placebo-controlled study. *The Journal of Clinical Psychiatry, 77*(12), e1610-e1617.

Ota, M., Wakabayashi, C., Sato, N., Hori, H., Hattori, K., Teraishi, T., & ... Kunugi, H. (2015). Effect of L-theanine on glutamatergic function in patients with schizophrenia. *Acta Neuropsychiatrica, 27*(5), 291-296.

Parsons Jr, W. (1964). *The effect of nicotinic acid on the liver. Evidence favoring functional alteration of enzymatic reactions without hepatocellular damage.* In R. Altshul, C. Thomas (Eds.) Niacin in Vascular Disorders and Hyperlipemia.

Patrick, R. P., & Ames, B. N. (2014). Vitamin D hormone regulates serotonin synthesis. Part 1: relevance for autism. *FASEB Journal*, 28(6), 2398-2413.

Patrick, R. P., & Ames, B. N. (2015). Vitamin D and the omega-3 fatty acids control serotonin synthesis and action, part 2: relevance for ADHD, bipolar disorder, schizophrenia, and impulsive behavior. *The FASEB Journal*, 29(6), 2207- 2222.

Pauling, L. (1974). On the orthomolecular environment of the mind: Orthomolecular theory. *The American Journal of Psychiatry*, 131(11), 1251-1257.

Pauling, L., Robinson, A., Oxley, S., Bergeson, M., Harris, A., Cary, P., ... Keaveny, I. (1973). *Vitamin C: New Biochemical and functional insights*. In D. Hawkins & L. Pauling (Eds.), Orthomolecular Psychiatry (W.H. Freeman, San Francisco 1973).

Prousky, J. (2006). *The orthomolecular treatment of schizophrenia*. Naturopathic Doctor News and Review. https://ndnr.com/neurology/the-orthomolecular-treatment-of-schizophrenia/.

Prousky, J. (2007, February/March). *The orthomolecular treatment of schizophrenia: A primer for clinicians*. Townsend Letter for Doctors & Patients.

Prousky, J. (2010). Understanding the serum vitamin B12 level and its implications for treating neuropsychiatric conditions: An Orthomolecular Perspective. *Journal of Orthomolecular Medicine*, 25(2).

Rapado-Castro, M., Berk, M., Venugopal, K., Bush, A. I., Dodd, S., & Dean, O. M. (2015). Towards stage specific treatments: effects of duration of illness on therapeutic response to adjunctive treatment with N-acetyl cysteine in schizophrenia. *Progress in Neuro-Psychopharmacology and Biological Psychiatry*, 57, 69-75.

Ritsner, M., Miodownik, C., Ratner, Y., Shleifer, T., Mar, M., Pintov, L., & Lerner, V. (2011). L-theanine relieves positive, activation, and anxiety symptoms in patients with schizophrenia and schizoaffective disorder: An 8-week, randomized, double-blind, placebo-controlled, 2-center study. *The Journal of Clinical Psychiatry*, 72(1), 34-42.

Saedisomeolia, A., Djalali, M., Moghadam, A. M., Ramezankhani, O., & Najmi, L. (2011). Folate and vitamin B12 status in schizophrenic patients. *Journal of Research in Medical Sciences*, 16(13), 437-441.

Sandyk, R., & Kanofsky, J. D. (1993). Vitamin C in the treatment of schizophrenia. *International Journal Of Neuroscience*, 68(1-2), 67-71.

Shirayama, Y., Obata, T., Matsuzawa, D., Nonaka, H., Kanazawa, Y., Yoshitome, E., & ... Iyo, M. (2010). Specific metabolites in the medial prefrontal cortex are associated with the neurocognitive deficits in schizophrenia: A preliminary study. *Neuroimage*, 49(3), 2783.

Smythies, J. (2002). The adrenochrome hypothesis of schizophrenia revisited. *Neurotoxicity Research*, 4(2), 147-150. https://doi.org/10.1080/10298420290015827.

Smythies, J. R. (1996). The role of ascorbate in brain: Therapeutic implications. *Journal of the Royal Society of Medicine*, 89(5), 241.

Song, X., Fan, X., Li, X., Zhang, W., Gao, J., Zhao, J., ... & Lv, L. (2014). Changes in pro-inflammatory cytokines and body weight during 6-month risperidone treatment in drug naive, first-episode schizophrenia. *Psychopharmacology*, 231(2), 319-325.

Suboticanec, K., Folnegović-Smalc, V., Korbar, M., Mestrović, B., & Buzina, R. (1990). Vitamin C status in chronic schizophrenia. *Biological Psychiatry*, 28(11), 959-966.

Orthomolecular treatment for schizophrenia

First principles

The four basic principles must be observed, i.e. shelter, nutrients, the doctor-patient relationship and orthomolecular treatment. The objective is complete recovery, which is defined here as the patient is: free of symptoms and signs; getting on well with family; getting on well with the community; and paying income tax or otherwise engaged in useful, productive and satisfying activities.

The fourth essential element of treatment is medical and includes the use of drugs as adjuncts and of course, orthomolecular methods.

When the four are combined, as we do in orthomolecular psychiatry, the recovery rate, when cases are treated early, should be close to 90%.

Orthomolecular treatment reinforces the natural ability of the body to heal itself when the level of stress is decreased.

Orthomolecular recovery rates in schizophrenia

I will not write about cures because the word cure has so many different meanings. And if patients are told they are cured they may assume that they no longer have to follow the program which got them well. It is a semantic problem. Every human suffers from pellagra but we are not sick because we all take enough B3 to prevent it from occurring.

I will write about recovery and recovery rates. This depends upon many factors such as how long the condition has been present, how it has been treated in the past and whether there is any brain damage.

For schizophrenia the recovery rates are as follows:

Very early or pre-schizophrenic patients: Often they will not need medication. If they are treated for at least one year, over 90% should be well.

Patients sick less than two years or who have been treated previously, have recovered but have relapsed: Treatment cures for two years should yield nearly 90% recovery rate

Patients sick up to ten years with intervals when they have been much better: Treatment up to ten years should recover over 50%.

Patients sick more that half their lifespan may need up to 20 years of treatment.

Almost all will be better, a few will be well but having lost so much out of life, they may never become well enough to meet the recovery criteria but they will be much more comfortable.

Treating schizophrenic patients is a long term commitment between patients, their families and the treating doctor. If every schizophrenic patient were diagnosed very early and treated promptly, nearly 90% would recover. The longer the disease has been present untreated, the greater the long-term harm to the patients.

Jonathan Prousky, ND
The Orthomolecular Treatment of Schizophrenia:
A Primer for Clinicians (Prousky, 2007)

Chronic patients required vitamin B3 treatment for five or more years in order to derive observable benefits (Hoffer, 1998; Hoffer 2001b).

Results are sometimes seen after the first two months," and sometimes three to six months are necessary before clinical benefits are observed (Hoffer, 2004).

Regardless of when the orthomolecular treatments begin to demonstrate their effectiveness, it is paramount that, once initiated, they are never discontinued.

Medications should likewise not be discontinued but, with the cooperation of the patient's psychiatrist, can be reduced very slowly over the course of many months to several years once the orthomolecular treatments are helping.

Abrupt cessation of atypical APDs will cause a relapse, as will, too much or too early of a decrease in medication.

The orthomolecular approach requires a tremendous amount of patience from the prescribing clinician, since results take a long time to materialize. Likewise, schizophrenic patients and their respective families and/or caregivers need to have the necessary patience and motivation to stay the course.

Expanding Hoffer's orthomolecular treatment of schizophrenia

Jonathan Prousky, ND, MSc, MA

The late Dr. Abram Hoffer always believed (and proved) that vitamin B3 was most essential in facilitating clinical improvement and recovery among patients with schizophrenia. Through meticulous clinical discovery and empirical research, he evolved his approach to schizophrenia treatment to include additional micronutrients, with optimal doses of vitamin B3, for the best possible clinical outcomes. Essentially, Dr. Hoffer's orthomolecular approach, as described in this book, included the following core micronutrient treatments: vitamin B3, vitamin C, high-dose B-complex vitamins, minerals (i.e., mainly zinc and manganese), and omega-3 essential fatty acids (Hoffer, 1998).

If Dr. Hoffer was alive today, he would use all available integrative orthomolecular treatments so that his patients would achieve greater capacities to live a normal life, or as near a normal life, as is possible.

Dr. Hoffer regrettably observed that schizophrenic patients become tranquilized as a result of their psychiatric medications, especially the antipsychotics, which create enormous dependency states associated with alarming brain-and body-based harms and complications (Prousky, 2013).

Full recoveries while taking orthomolecular substances, or even benefiting from other helpful interventions, are less likely to happen as long as schizophrenic patients remain loaded-up on their cocktails of psychiatric medications. Patients will only improve once the daily burden of psychiatric medication is reduced over time.

Schizophrenia psychosis and the tranquilizer psychosis

Dr. Hoffer knew these complex clinical issues extremely well and discussed them in detail (Hoffer, 1994). When patients are becoming psychotic, or have manifested all manner of signs and symptoms of psychosis, a lot of unwanted attention happens.

Any normal individual would find psychotic manifestations intolerable, though the individual experiencing psychosis does not usually have the necessary insight to feel the same way.

Antipsychotic medications are needed to bring quick stability to any individual experiencing this type of profound mental distress. The unfortunate problem is that when the antipsychotic medications are used to stabilize psychotic patients, patients diagnosed with schizophrenia often remain ill for the long-term, as long they are maintained on the same (or even higher) doses of psychiatric medication.

In Dr. Hoffer's words, "the entire schizophrenic psychosis has been replaced by the tranquilizer psychosis" (p. 13).

The following table shows the contrast between the schizophrenia psychosis and the tranquilizer psychosis that develops when schizophrenic patients are medicated over the long-term without ever having their daily doses of antipsychotics reduced.

Schizophrenic psychosis compared to the tranquilizer psychosis

Adapted from Hoffer (2004, p. 6); used with permission.

Signs and Symptoms	Schizophrenia Psychosis	Tranquilizer Psychosis
Perception	Voices	Not as intense, or eliminated
	Visions	Same
	Illusions	Same
Thought Disorder	Content: Paranoid	Not as intense
	Delusional	Same or less
	Ideas of reference	Same or less
	Process: Blocking	Not as intense
	Memory	Same or worse
	Concentration	Same or worse
Mood	Depression	Same
	Agitation	Less
	Anxiety	Less
	Apathy	More
	Disinterest	More
Behavior	Abnormal persistent activity and/or inappropriate activity	Subdued, slowed, sedentary
Physical Toxicity	None	Tardive dyskinesia, tardive dystonia, and/or parkinsonism. Nausea. Brain damage. Weight gain. Blood sugar problems, or diabetes. Sexual dysfunction

The rationale for giving antipsychotic medication is to assist patients with the process of recovery, which is exactly what they do rather quickly, by decreasing the intensity of signs and symptoms. However, as Dr. Hoffer noted:

But as the patient begins this process and their symptoms decrease in intensity and frequency, their physiology, which must also become more and more normal, begins to respond to the drugs as if they were well, i.e. it makes them sick. They produce the tranquilizer psychosis. The tranquilizer psychosis is iatrogenic, induced by the doctor who has prescribed the drug. It causes both mental and physical symptoms (Hoffer, 1994, pp. 12-13).

If schizophrenic patients have their antipsychotic medications reduced, but nothing more, the original psychosis will invariably return, necessitating going back on antipsychotic medication. The schizophrenic patient will then oscillate between the schizophrenia and tranquilizer psychosis, when off and on antipsychotic medication respectively (Hoffer, 1994).

Recovery is possible with integrative orthomolecular treatment

To remedy this clinical conundrum, Dr. Hoffer integrated the usual care involving antipsychotic medication (and other psychiatric medications) with an orthomolecular approach, as soon as it was clinically possible. Unlike other psychiatrists, he was able to reduce the daily doses of antipsychotic medication, and see the schizophrenic patients under his care thrive and live life in ways that other psychiatrists did not even believe was possible.

Schizophrenic patients should consider beginning with vitamin B3 (my clinical preference is niacin), B-complex, vitamin C, and omega-3 essential fatty acids in the optimal daily doses described in this book.

Additional orthomolecular treatments that go beyond Dr. Hoffer's foundational approach should be considered to further improve clinical outcomes. I have no doubt that Dr. Hoffer would have incorporated many of the additional orthomolecular treatments discussed below based on their safety and therapeutic efficacy.

Amino acid therapies: N-acetylcysteine (NAC), L-lysine, and L-theanine

NAC

NAC is a precursor to glutathione, which is a natural antioxidant produced in the body. Glutathione is presumed to be deficient in the brains of schizophrenic patients (Sansone & Sansone, 2011). NAC has been shown to increase blood glutathione levels (Lavoie et al., 2007), and modulate the glutamatergic system (Dean, Giorlando, & Berk, 2011). A dysfunctional glutamatergic system has been linked to psychosis and clinical deterioration. For instance, drugs like ketamine and phencyclidine disrupt the glutamatergic system and cause psychotic symptoms that mimic schizophrenia (Marsman et al., 2013).

A clinical trial added NAC (1,000 mg twice daily over 24 weeks) to medicated patients with chronic schizophrenia (Berk et al., 2008). Compared to placebo, the patients treated with NAC had improvements in their negative symptoms, global function, and akathisia (i.e., a feeling of inner restlessness and inability to stay still). The improvements ceased within one month of discontinuing the orthomolecule. These improvements are noteworthy since all these patients were ill for an average of 12 years, and more than 60% were taking clozapine.

A similar study showed statistically-significant improvements in negative symptoms among chronic schizophrenic patients given NAC (up to 2,000 mg/day) in combination with risperidone (taking up to 6 mg/day; Farokhnia et al., 2013).

A double-blind study with patients with chronic schizophrenia provided NAC (1,200 mg/day) as add-on treatment along with antipsychotic medication (Sepehrmanesh, Heidary, Akasheh, Akbari, & Heidary, 2018). At the conclusion of the 12 week trial, patients taking NAC had improvements in positive, negative, and general and total psychopathology symptoms. Cognitive improvements were also observed in attention, short-term and working memory, executive functioning, and speed of processing. The frequency of adverse effects were not significantly different between the add-on NAC and medication only groups.

In a 12-month clinical trial, NAC (3,600 mg/day) was given to schizophrenic patients in the early phase of their illness to assess its impacts upon cognition and symptoms (Breier et al., 2018). The use of NAC improved the overall status of the patients, as well as negative symptoms, and disorganized thoughts. The results of this study confirmed many prior clinical outcomes that have been attributed to the use of NAC.

Other studies have evaluated some of the mechanisms that have been attributed to NAC's therapeutic effects. A study involving 19 schizophrenic patients showed that NAC (2,400 mg/day) was able to modulate the levels of glutamate in a particular brain area known as the anterior cingulate cortex (McQeen et al., 2018). Another study on early psychosis patients demonstrated that NAC (2,700 mg/day) for 6 months resulted in increased functional connectivity within the cingulate cortex (Mullier et al., 2019). The alterations within the cingulate cortex were presumed to "impact the connectivity between other brain subnetworks and connectivity of other functional systems" (Mullier et al., 2019, p. 485). In other words, by helping the glutamatergic system in one brain area, NAC might productively influence other brain areas implicated in schizophrenia.

NAC can be safely combined with atypical antipsychotic medication and may also benefit akathisia. NAC can be combined with all classes of psychiatric medication. The daily dose lies somewhere between 2,000–3,600 mg/day. The only limiting factor is that some patients experience gastrointestinal symptoms (Dean, Giorlando, & Berk, 2011), such as unpleasant nausea or stomach upset, making the amino acid difficult to tolerate. It needs to be taken away from food for maximal therapeutic efficacy.

Lysine

By inhibiting arginine transport, the supplemental use of lysine (L-lysine) is believed to decrease nitric oxide levels, and reduce symptoms of schizophrenia (i.e., the "nitric oxide dysregulation hypothesis of schizophrenia;" (Wass et al., 2011).

In a clinical study lysine (6,000 mg mixed with juice or a soft drink) once daily resulted in increased lysine blood concentrations in 8 out of 10 patients, and decreased in positive symptoms. The use of lysine did not perturb the levels of other amino acids that were tested. However, positive symptoms, such as delusions and suspiciousness/persecution improved. Further data analysis showed that the reductions in positive symptoms could not be solely attributed to that of the lysine supplementation.

Lysine also improved problem-solving capacity and cognitive flexibility. Two of the patients that responded noted decreases in their auditory hallucinations when on lysine, which returned when the study ended because they stopped taking the amino acid.

One patient reported improved attention while taking lysine, while another noted improved mental stability and memory capacity that continued for several weeks after the trial ended. Overall, these results demonstrated that lysine improved cognitive function, and possibly reduced positive symptoms.

In another trial, lysine (3,000 mg twice daily) was administered for 8 weeks (Zeinoddini et al., 2014). There were significant reductions in both negative symptoms, and general psychopathology subscale scores.

Improvement in negative symptoms is an important treatment target since they are often associated with progressive disability and cannot be effectively treated by antipsychotic medication (Zeinoddini et al., 2014).

Improvement in general psychopathology subscale scores reflect improvements in cognitive deficits, such as disorientation, poor attention, lack of insight, and active social avoidance (Shankar & Nate, 2007).

The findings by Wass et al (2011) from the first study were important since all the patients had been ill for a duration of 3-29 years, and were on various combinations of atypical antipsychotic medications (6 of 10 patients were taking at least two atypical antipsychotic medications).

The findings by (Zeinoddini et al., 2014) from the second study were also important since the trial involved many more patients, and showed a different spectrum of therapeutic effects when lysine was given to patients on risperidone.

No significant adverse effects were associated with lysine treatment in both trials, except transient gastrointestinal problems (Wass et al., 2011). The daily dose of lysine should be 6,000 mg given in powder form mixed with juice or capsules to be swallowed, and needs to be taken away from food. Lysine can be safely combined with all classes of psychiatric medication.

Theanine

Theanine (L-theanine) possesses several important mechanisms of action that include the following: being able to readily pass the blood-brain barrier; possessing gamma-aminobutyric acid (GABA) agonist (i.e., calming) effects; protecting against glutamate neurotoxicity; stimulating the release of nerve growth factor; modulating brain-derived neurotrophic factor (BDNF); and possessing antioxidant activity (Ritsner et al., 2011).

In a clinical trial, theanine or placebo was given to schizophrenic and schizoaffective disorder patients as add-on treatment with antipsychotic medication (Ritsner et al., 2011). Sixty patients were randomized to placebo or theanine (400 mg/day) for 8 weeks, but only 40 patients completed the trial.

The beneficial effects from theanine began at the second week of the trial. Theanine was associated with significant reductions in positive symptoms, general psychopathology scores, and anxiety. Another measurement showed theanine to be associated with a reduction in activation factor (i.e., a marker of hostility and aggression.

A subsequent analysis (Miodownik et al., 2011) evaluated blood levels of various neurochemicals from the same 40 patients that completed the above-mentioned trial. The analysis showed that the beneficial effects of theanine were associated with circulating levels of BDNF, and the cortisol-to-dehydroepiandrosterone (DHEA) ratio. BDNF is a protein found in the brain and spinal cord that helps neurons (brain cells) to survive, grow, build better connections with other neurons, and assist with learning and long-term memory.

The cortisol-to-DHEA ratio is a marker of stress, and smaller ratios or lower amounts of cortisol relative to higher levels of DHEA improve a person's ability to cope with adversity, and increase resilience.

In another study, theanine was given to patients with chronic schizophrenia (Ota et al., 2015), The aim of the study was to assess the therapeutic properties of theanine, and to determine if they are mediated by changes in the glutamatergic system.

Seventeen patients were given theanine (250 mg/day) in addition to their regular antipsychotic medication for the 8 weeks. Theanine was shown to improve overall functional status, and to improve sleep quality. Brain imaging showed that theanine stabilized the glutamatergic concentration in the brain, which was presumed to be the mechanism responsible for these observed therapeutic changes.

A combination study utilizing the hormone, pregnenolone with theanine as adjuncts to antipsychotic therapy will be discussed later in the hormone section (Kardashev, Ratner, & Ritsner, 2018).

I have not observed any adverse effects from the therapeutic use of theanine. The daily dose should be at least 400–450 mg. It is best taken at bedtime since it can also assist with sleep. It can be combined with any class of psychiatric medication as an augmentation strategy.

Broad-spectrum micronutrient treatment

A broad-spectrum approach using micronutrients has been shown to benefit schizophrenic patients.

In a study by Mehl-Madrona and Mainguy (2017), large doses of broad-spectrum micronutrients (i.e., comprised of vitamins and minerals; Figure 1, p.4) was given to patients with a confirmed psychotic disorder diagnosis. Nineteen of the participants were given the broad-spectrum micronutrients (4 capsules twice daily) added to their psychiatric medications compared to 59 patients that remained only on their respective psychiatric medications.

All participants were evaluated by various measures over the course of 24 months. The clinical outcomes for both groups were similar until 15 months though the group of patients taking the add-on broad-spectrum micronutrients needed significantly less antipsychotic medication by that time.

At 15 to 24 months the group of patients taking the add-on broad-spectrum micronutrients showed significantly fewer symptoms. Another notable finding was that the group of patients taking the add- on broad-spectrum micronutrients needed much less psychiatric medication for their ongoing stability compared to the medication-only group of patients.

Lastly, the group of patients taking the add-on broad-spectrum micronutrients experienced fewer adverse effects compared to patients only taking psychiatric medication.

Given all the potential biochemical problems that have been linked to schizophrenia, it is not surprising that a combination of micronutrients would result in beneficial clinical outcomes. By raising the level of micronutrient concentrations within the body and central nervous system (CNS), there would likely be corrections to the various neurochemical issues that have been associated with schizophrenia pathology, such as glutathione deficiency in the brain, and glutamatergic dysfunction.

Hormonal therapies: pregnenolone, DHEA, and thyroid

The neurosteroid pregnenolone has been shown to enhance learning and memory in rodents, and has been hypothesized to attenuate glutamatergic dysfunction (Marx et al., 2009).

Both pregnenolone and DHEA modulate neuronal excitability, synaptic plasticity, and the stress response; all of which has been implicated in mood regulation and cognitive performance (Ritsner et al., 2010).

Unfortunately, clinical trials evaluating therapeutic doses of DHEA among patients with schizophrenia are sparse. Pregnenolone, on the other hand, has been subjected to several clinical trials.

The use of pregnenolone was studied to determine if it could improve cognitive and negative symptoms in patients with schizophrenia or schizoaffective disorder on stable doses of antipsychotic medication (Marx et al., 2009).

Pregnenolone (500 mg/day) reduced negative symptoms, and showed potential as a treatment for cognitive symptoms.

Both pregnenolone and DHEA were evaluated as add-on treatment to patients with schizophrenia and schizoaffective disorder (Ritsner et al., 2010). Patients given 30 mg/day of pregnenolone had significant reductions in positive symptoms, and reductions in extrapyramidal side effects (EPS) that commonly make patients look as though they have Parkinson's disease (i.e., parkinsonism).

Pregnenolone was also associated with improvements in attention and working memory performance. Patients on DHEA (400 mg/day) showed greater improvements in EPS compared to placebo. The main conclusions from this trial were that low-dose pregnenolone (30 mg/day) demonstrated benefits on positive symptoms, EPS, and cognitive function.

In another clinical trial lasting 8 weeks, pregnenolone (50 mg/day) or placebo was given to patients with recent-onset schizophrenia and schizoaffective disorder (Ritsner, Bawakny, & Kreinin, 2014).

Compared to placebo, pregnenolone reduced negative symptoms, particularly on blunted affect, avolition, and anhedonia domain scores. The benefits of pregnenolone were more pronounced among patients that were not also taking mood stabilizers.

A randomized controlled trial lasting 8 weeks assessed both theanine (400 mg/day) and pregnenolone (50 mg/day) among patients with schizophrenia and schizoaffective disorder (Kardashev,

Ratner, & Ritsner, 2015). Patients on the combination of pregnenolone and theanine had significant improvements in negative symptoms, such as blunted affect, alogia, and anhedonia Similarly, the combination of pregnenolone and theanine reduced anxiety scores, including domains of anxious mood, tension, and cardiovascular symptoms.

Other trials on pregnenolone have been done. A trial that involved patients with recent-onset schizophrenia and schizoaffective disorder showed that pregnenolone (50 mg/day) significantly reduced deficits in visual and sustained attention, and in executive functioning (Kreinin, Bawakny, & Ritsner, 2017).

A trial on women with chronic schizophrenia showed that pregnenolone (50 mg/day) in addition to risperidone resulted in changes in positive symptoms and general psychopathology (Kashani et al., 2017).

The use of pregnenolone and DHEA were not shown to produce adverse effects different from placebo in one of the clinical trials described previously (Ritsner et al., 2010). All the other trials (Marx et al., 2009; Ritsner et al., 2014; Kardashev, Ratner, & Ritsner, 2015; Kreinin, Bawakny, & Ritsner, 2017; and Kashani et al., 2017 did not find any significant differences between pregnenolone and placebo in terms of adverse effects.

The reader of this chapter is recommended to review the paper by Ritsner (2011) for a more comprehensive understanding of these neurosteroids and schizophrenia, including possible adverse effects.

DHEA did not impact any symptoms of schizophrenia from the cited trials though it helped with EPS. However, an inverse association was found between higher blood levels of DHEA, and/or higher blood DHEA-to-cortisol ratios and lower schizophrenic symptoms among 17 medicated chronic inpatients (Harris, Wolkowitz, & Reus, 2001).

The dose of DHEA used to treat schizophrenia symptoms is not known though 400 mg/day was used by Ritsner et al., (2010), and was not associated with any adverse effects. The dose of pregnenolone that produced consistent beneficial effects among patients with schizophrenia was usually 50 mg/day though a dose as high as 500 mg/day was also shown to produce therapeutic benefits (Marx et al., 2009).

Thyroid hormones, which can function as neurotransmitters like pregnenolone and DHEA, are essential to the proper development of the CNS and assist with the following:

1. neuronal myelination;
2. proinflammatory responses in the brain;
3. the regulation of dopaminergic, serotonergic, glutamatergic, and GABAergic systems;
4. the synthesis and regulation of brain receptors; and
5. treatment response (Seddigh, Azarnik, & Keshavarz-Akhlaghi, 2015).

There does seem to be a relationship between thyroid status and schizophrenia. In one study, some 36% of chronic schizophrenic patients were found to have abnormal thyroid tests even though their actual thyroid status was considered to be clinically normal (Sim, Chong, Chan, & Lum, 2002).

Another study showed that 25% of chronic schizophrenic patients had evidence of thyroid dysfunction (Themeli, Aliko, & Hashorva, 2011). A report even showed that thyroid function is often impaired as a consequence of simply being on psychiatric medication (Vickery, Mathews, & Vickery, 2019).

Thus, there is reason to believe that abnormal thyroid results are associated with greater symptoms among schizophrenic patients. These effects may be due to the mental illness itself, and/or as a consequence of being treated with psychiatric medication.

Dr. Hoffer even reported that some patients with schizophrenia benefited when prescription desiccated thyroid extract (DTE) was added to a treatment plan involving usual care with antipsychotic medication and optimal daily doses of niacin (Hoffer, 2001a).

He reviewed the literature on this topic, and reported on 12 patients in which the addition of large doses of DTE resulted in therapeutic improvements among 9 of them. One of his patients had previously been admitted 16 times to the University Hospital, had almost normalized from the addition of DTE, and became free of auditory hallucinations.

Dr. Hoffer observed that patients with schizophrenia could tolerate very large doses of DTE, and needed them because adrenochrome and/or other factors (e.g., micronutrient insufficiency, aging, excessive oxidation, and liver and kidney disease) undermined or even antagonized the production of the thyroid hormones, such as thyroxine (T4), and the more active thyroid hormone known as triiodothyronine (T3).

There is even a published case demonstrating symptom remission from thyroid medication in a patient taking clozapine (600 mg/day) with persistent schizophrenic symptoms (Seddigh et al., 2015). When the patient was given 100 mcg of T4 medication, her hallucinations and delusions completely went away by 2 weeks, and her social relations also improved. Then the T4 medication was stopped, and 3 weeks later her psychosis once again reappeared as evidenced by the presence of hallucinations and delusions. The patient resumed 100 mcg of T4 medication in addition to her regular doses of clozapine, and the psychosis once again remitted after 2 weeks, and did not return over the course of 12 months of follow-up care.

Throughout this entire treatment period, the patient's thyroid status was normal, and was never diagnostically abnormal even before taking prescribed thyroid medication. This represents a case of normal thyroid function in a schizophrenic patient that responded therapeutically to thyroid medication.

Given Dr. Hoffer's clinical experience, and cases such as the one described above, consideration ought to be given to prescription thyroid medication to further support recovery among schizophrenic patients. Dr. Hoffer's usual maintenance dose was 5 grains of DTE daily. One grain (65 mg) of DTE contains 38 mcg of T4 and 9 mcg of T3 (Hoang, Olsen, Mai, Clyde, & Shakir, 2013). Personally, I would not provide schizophrenic patients with such large doses of DTE. Rather, and based on appropriate thyroid testing, I would likely begin with 1/2 grain of DTE (or 50 mcg of T4) and proceed slowly while also monitoring the patient's clinical response, the blood levels of thyroid hormones.

Improving the current situation

Poor adherence to psychiatric medication is believed to explain frequent relapses following treatment, and is regrettably associated with clinical deterioration and declining functionality over time (Lewis & Lieberman, 2000). So, too, is the tranquilizer psychosis that was described earlier (Hoffer, 1994; Hoffer, 2004). These issues most certainly present serious problems for schizophrenic patients.

On the one hand, schizophrenic patients are often loaded-up on several psychiatric medications, which they have been told will be needed for the rest of their lives as a result of the expected chronicity of the mental illness.

On the other hand, many schizophrenic patients detest how psychiatric medications make them feel, and so they often discontinue them abruptly with hopes of not needing them any longer. This begets the vicious cycle discussed earlier that cycles patients between the schizophrenia psychosis and the tranquilizer psychosis.

When patients are given effective orthomolecular treatment the vicious cycle of going on and off psychiatric medication is halted.

Schizophrenic patients need to be on an integrative orthomolecular approach for at least 2-6 months before some of the benefits are observed. Patients will usually report improvements in energy, motivation, anxiety, and/or mood over the course of 2-6 months.

If patients are stable at 2-6 months and have tolerated the orthomolecular approach well, the daily dose of antipsychotic medication can be slowly reduced.

The process of slowly lowering the antipsychotic medication along with adjustments to the orthomolecular approach should continue until patients are maintained on the lowest dose of antipsychotic medication they require. This also eases and sometimes eliminates the tranquilizer psychosis, allowing schizophrenic patients to remain stable and well on less psychiatric medication.

This approach works best for new-onset schizophrenic patients, but also shows durable clinical benefits when given to chronic patients with the illness (Hoffer, 1994). The orthomolecular approach should be maintained throughout the patient's life so that the therapeutic benefits remain, and this should be in concert with proper and regular clinician oversight.

Putting it all together

When reviewing the potential therapeutic benefits from the above-mentioned orthomolecules, it appears that they can moderate psychotic symptoms, and improve cognitive function. This information has been summarized in the following table.

Symptom-moderating effects of orthomolecular substances not part of Dr. Hoffer's foundational orthomolecular treatment approach

Potentially improves positive symptoms	Potentially improves negative symptoms	Potentially improves cognitive function
• NAC • Lysine • Theanine • Broad-Spectrum micro-nutrients • Thyroid hormone • pregnenolone • DHEA (requires further study)	• NAC • Lysine • Broad-Spectrum micro-nutrients • pregnenolone	• NAC • Lysine • pregnenolone

no longer incurred any mental health hospitalization costs, except needing to pay approximately $720.00 per year for the broad-spectrum micronutrient supplement.

It would seem negligent when patients aren't advised to integrate an orthomolecular approach with customary care. This chapter both highlighted the tremendous value that the orthomolecular approach affords to schizophrenic patients in terms of regaining the quality of their lives back, but also the immediate urgency to do so and make the current situation better.

In conclusion

The potential savings to our healthcare system would likely be substantial if this approach were to become "the routine" way schizophrenia is managed.

Dr. Hoffer always described the tremendous cost-savings to the healthcare system, and the countless patient lives that were spared from interminable misery, from using the orthomolecular approach.

A study did evaluate the healthcare savings that resulted in a patient that used broad-spectrum micronutrients to control the chronicity of her disabling psychotic disorder diagnosis (Kaplan, Isaranuwatchal, & Hoch, 2017).

Her annual mental health hospitalization costs while under conventional treatment only averaged $59,864 over 5 years (1997-2001), and peaked to $140,000 at one point. Since integrating with broad-spectrum micronutrients, she

References

Berk, M., Copolov, D., Dean, O., Lu, K., Jeavons, S., Schapkaitz, I., . . . Bush, A. I. (2008). N-acetyl cysteine as a glutathione precursor for schizophrenia—A double-blind, randomized, placebo-controlled Trial. *Biological Psychiatry*, 64(5), 361-368.

Breier, A., Liffick, E., Hummer, T. A., Vohs, J. L., Yang, Z., Mehdiyoun, N. F., . . . Francis, M. M. (2018). Effects of 12-month, double-blind N-acetyl cysteine on symptoms, cognition and brain morphology in early phase schizophrenia spectrum disorders. *Schizophrenia Research*, 199, 395-402.

Dean, O., Giorlando, F., & Berk, M. (2011). N-acetylcysteine in psychiatry: Current therapeutic evidence and potential mechanisms of action. *Journal of Psychiatry & Neuroscience*, 36(2), 78-86.

Farokhnia, M., Azarkolah, A., Adinehfar, F., Khodaie-Ardakani, M., Hosseini, S., Yekehtaz, H., . . . Akhondzadeh, S. (2013). N-acetylcysteine as an adjunct to risperidone for treatment of negative symptoms in patients with chronic schizophrenia. *Clinical Neuropharmacology*, 36(6), 185-192.

Harris, D. S., Wolkowitz, O. M., & Reus, V. I. (2001). Movement disorder, memory, psychiatric symptoms and serum DHEA levels in schizophrenic and schizoaffective Patients. *World Journal of Biological Psychiatry*, 2(2), 99-102.

Hoang, T. D., Olsen, C. H., Mai, V. Q., Clyde, P. W., & Shakir, M. K. (2013). Desiccated thyroid extract compared with levothyroxine in the treatment of hypothyroidism: A randomized, double-blind, crossover study. *Journal of Clinical Endocrinology & Metabolism*, *98*(5), 1982-1990.

Hoffer, A. (1994). Chronic schizophrenic patients treated ten years or more. *Journal of Orthomolecular Medicine*, *9*, 7-37.

Hoffer, A. (1998). *Vitamin B3 & schizophrenia* (pp. 94-121). Kingston, ON: Quarry Press, Inc.

Hoffer, A. (2001). Thyroid and schizophrenia. *Journal of Orthomolecular Medicine*, *16*(4), 205-212.

Hoffer, A. (2004). Atypical anti-psychotics create dependency disorders. *Journal of Orthomolecular Medicine*, *19*, 3-10.

Kaplan, B. J., Isaranuwatchai, W., & Hoch, J. S. (2017). Hospitalization cost of conventional psychiatric care compared to broad-spectrum micronutrient treatment: Literature review and case study of adult psychosis. *International Journal of Mental Health Systems*, *11*(1).

Kardashev, A., Ratner, Y., & Ritsner, M. S. (2018). Add-on pregnenolone with L-theanine to antipsychotic therapy relieves negative and anxiety symptoms of schizophrenia: An 8-week, randomized, double-blind, placebo-controlled trial. *Clinical Schizophrenia & Related Psychoses*, *12*(1), 31-41.

Kashani, L., Shams, N., Moazen-Zadeh, E., Karkhaneh-Yousefi, M., Sadighi, G., Khodaie-Ardakani, M., . . . Akhondzadeh, S. (2017). Pregnenolone as an adjunct to risperidone for treatment of women with schizophrenia: A randomized double-blind placebo-controlled clinical trial. *Journal of Psychiatric Research*, *94*, 70-77.

Kreinin, A., Bawakny, N., & Ritsner, M. S. (2017). Adjunctive pregnenolone ameliorates the cognitive deficits in recent-onset schizophrenia: An 8-week, randomized, double-blind, placebo-controlled trial. *Clinical Schizophrenia & Related Psychoses*, *10*(4), 201-210.

Lavoie, S., Murray, M. M., Deppen, P., Knyazeva, M. G., Berk, M., Boulat, O., . . . Do, K. Q. (2007). Glutathione precursor, N-Acetyl-cysteine, improves mismatch negativity in schizophrenia patients. *Neuropsychopharmacology*, *33*(9), 2187-2199.

Lewis, D. A., & Lieberman, J. A. (2000). Catching up on schizophrenia. *Neuron*, *28*(2), 325-334.

Marsman, A., Heuvel, M. P., Klomp, D. W., Kahn, R. S., Luijten, P. R., & Pol, H. E. (2013). Glutamate in schizophrenia: A focused review and meta-analysis of 1H-MRS studies. *Schizophrenia Bulletin*, *39*(1), 120-129.

Marx, C. E., Keefe, R. S., Buchanan, R. W., Hamer, R. M., Kilts, J. D., Bradford, D. W., . . . Shampine, L. J. (2009). Proof-of-concept trial with the neurosteroid pregnenolone targeting cognitive and negative symptoms in schizophrenia. *Neuropsychopharmacology*, *34*(8), 1885-1903.

Mcqueen, G., Lally, J., Collier, T., Zelaya, F., Lythgoe, D. J., Barker, G. J., . . . Egerton, A. (2018). Effects of N-acetylcysteine on brain glutamate levels and resting perfusion in schizophrenia. *Psychopharmacology*, *235*(10), 3045-3054.

Mehl-Madrona, L., & Mainguy, B. (2017). Adjunctive treatment of psychotic disorders with micronutrients. *Journal of Alternative and Complementary Medicine*, *23*(7), 526-533.

Miodownik, C., Maayan, R., Ratner, Y., Lerner, V., Pintov, L., Mar, M., . . . Ritsner, M. S. (2011). Serum levels of brain-derived neurotrophic factor and cortisol to sulfate of dehydroepiandrosterone molar ratio associated with clinical response to L-theanine as augmentation of antipsychotic therapy in schizophrenia and schizoaffective disorder patients. *Clinical Neuropharmacology*, *34*(4), 155-160.

Mullier, E., Roine, T., Griffa, A., Xin, L., Baumann, P. S., Klauser, P., . . . Hagmann, P. (2019). N-acetyl-cysteine supplementation improves functional connectivity within the cingulate cortex in early psychosis: A pilot study. *International Journal of Neuropsychopharmacology*, *22*(8), 478-487.

Ota, M., Wakabayashi, C., Sato, N., Hori, H., Hattori, K., Teraishi, T., . . . Kunugi, H. (2015). Effect of L-theanine on glutamatergic function in patients with schizophrenia. *Acta Neuropsychiatrica*, *27*(5), 291-296.

Prousky, J. (2013). Orthomolecular psychiatric treatments are preferable to mainstream psychiatric drugs: A rational analysis. *Journal of Orthomolecular Medicine*, *28*(1), 17-32.

Ritsner, M. S., Bawakny, H., & Kreinin, A. (2014). Pregnenolone treatment reduces severity of negative symptoms in recent-onset schizophrenia: An 8-week, double-blind, randomized add-on two-center trial. *Psychiatry and Clinical Neurosciences*, *68*(6), 432-440.

Ritsner, M. S., Gibel, A., Shleifer, T., Boguslavsky, I., Zayed, A., Maayan, R., . . . Lerner, V. (2010). Pregnenolone and dehydroepiandrosterone as an adjunctive treatment in schizophrenia and schizoaffective disorder. *Journal of Clinical Psychiatry*, *71*(10), 1351-1362.

Ritsner, M. S., Miodownik, C., Ratner, Y., Shleifer, T., Mar, M., Pintov, L., & Lerner, V. (2011). L-theanine relieves positive, activation, and anxiety symptoms in patients with schizophrenia and schizoaffective disorder: An 8-week, randomized, double-blind, placebo-controlled, 2-center study. *Journal of Clinical Psychiatry*, *72*(1), 34-42.

Sansone, R. A., & Sansone, L. A. (2011). Getting a knack for NAC: N-acetyl-cysteine. *Innovations in Clinical Neuroscience*, *8*, 10-14.

Seddigh, R., Azarnik, S., & Keshavarz-Akhlaghi, A. (2015). Levothyroxine augmentation in clozapine resistant schizophrenia: A case report and review. *Case Reports in Psychiatry*, 2015, 1-4.

Sepehrmanesh, Z., Heidary, M., Akasheh, N., Akbari, H., & Heidary, M. (2018). Therapeutic effect of adjunctive N-acetyl cysteine (NAC) on symptoms of chronic schizophrenia: A double-blind, randomized clinical trial. *Progress in Neuro-Psychopharmacology and Biological Psychiatry*, *82*, 289-296.

Sim, K., Chong, S. A., Chan, Y. H., & Lum, W. M. (2002). Thyroid dysfunction in chronic schizophrenia within a state psychiatric hospital. *Annals of the Academy of Medicine*, *31*(5), 641–644.

Themeli, Y., Aliko, I., & Hashorva, A. (2011). P03-345 - Thyroid dysfunction in chronic schizophrenia in Albania. *European Psychiatry*, *26*(Suppl. 1), 1515.

Vickery, P. B., Mathews, A., & Vickery, S. B. (2019). Effects of psychotropic medications on thyroid function. *Current Psychiatry*, *18*(1), 61-63.

Wass, C., Klamer, D., Katsarogiannis, E., Pålsson, E., Svensson, L., Fejgin, K., ... Rembeck, B. (2011). L-lysine as adjunctive treatment in patients with schizophrenia: A single-blinded, randomized, cross-over pilot study. *BMC Medicine*, *9*(1). Retrieved from https://www.ncbi.nlm.nih.gov/pmc/articles/PMC3094237/pdf/1741-7015-9-40.pdf.

Zeinoddini, A., Ahadi, M., Farokhnia, M., Rezaei, F., Tabrizi, M., & Akhondzadeh, S. (2014). L-lysine as an adjunct to risperidone in patients with chronic schizophrenia: A double-blind, placebo-controlled, randomized Trial. *Journal of Psychiatric Research*, *59*, 125-131.

Legacy chapter

Segments from Dr. Hoffer's original book have been republished in this chapter to retain a record and provide more context, to his writings and work with schizophrenia and other mental illnesses.

Common questions about schizophrenia treatment

Q. What if my patient shows a very good response in a few months and then, while remaining on the same program, stops responding or relapses?

A. Usually this means that the dose of vitamin B3 has to be increased. If the starting dose was 1 g after each of three meals, it should be increased to 1.5 g three times daily or even 2 g. Occasionally the dose will need to be increased to 4 to 5 g, taken three times daily.

Q. My patient has been well for several years and wants to cut back on some of the vitamins?

A. This can be done, but very slowly. If there is any evidence of relapse such as increased fatigue and depression, the dose should be increased. If the patients can not afford all the program, the most important nutrient is vitamin B3 and it should always be continued.

Q. When should the medication be decreased?

A. The objective is for the patient to be well and free of side effects. This is achievable if the dose of medication is so low that there are only positive effects and no side effects. A few patients may need tiny doses of anti-psychotic medication such as risperidone 1 mg daily. Because these modern drugs are addictive and have made the patients depend on them it is very difficult to decrease the dose without a surge of serious withdrawal side effects. The best indication of when to decrease the dose is when patients are made too drowsy, have problems getting up in the morning and have concentration problems. Then the drug is decreased very slowly, perhaps by no more than ten percent of the dose being taken. After each dose change one should wait up to one month before decreasing the dose again. Older drugs such as haldol are not addictive and they can be decreased more rapidly without the same serious withdrawal side effects.

Q. What do I do if the patient having been well for some time starts to relapse.

A. Do your best to keep them out of any psychiatric ward unless there is no alternative. Their relapse will surely accelerate when all the nutrients are stopped. Your patient should demand that the nutrients be continued in hospital. If they can avoid admission you should increase the B3 (if it has been decreased) and can resume any medication using the usual indications.

Q. Can I treat young schizophrenic patients the same way?

A. The treatment is essentially the same. But if they are diagnosed early in most cases they will not need medication and this is a great advantage. The dose of nutrients is not related to body mass or to age. Very young patients can tolerate these doses as well as older patients.

Q. What about dual diagnoses especially schizophrenia and any of the addictions?

A. Many years ago David Hawkins, one of the pioneers in orthomolecular psychiatry, reported that the only treatment that had ever helped the alcoholic schizophrenic patients was the use of niacin, and the use of orthomolecular therapy. But his patients were also in Alcoholics Anonymous. Before he began to use niacin not one of these patients did well. If the schizophrenia came under some type of control, they would start drinking and would once more relapse into their schizophrenia. About five percent of these patients have both diagnoses. Dr. Russ Smith, in charge of a large hospital in Detroit specializing in the treatment of alcoholism found that adding niacin was the most important single treatment. And even with alcoholic patients who did not want to stop drinking but agreed to take niacin at the same time, he found that after several years many of them slowly decreased their alcoholic intake and eventually stopped. The alcoholic schizophrenic should be treated for both conditions but it is essential that they stop drinking and the best way is to encourage them to join Alcoholics Anonymous.

Schizophrenic patients may also be addicted to the drugs used to treat them. With the introduction of the modern atypical antipsychotics we are witnessing a new problem. Going off these drugs is more difficult than the older drugs such as haldol and chlorpromazine. With modern drugs even a ten percent decrease in dose will, within hours, cause severe withdrawal as if they were suddenly taken off heroin. As these patients did not voluntarily become addicted to these drugs, which were forced upon them by modern psychiatry, it is more appropriate to call them drug dependent. It is very important to withdraw these modern drugs very slowly and carefully in order to deal with their massive addicting properties.

Q. What if my patient has Hepatitis C? Can he use niacin or niacinamide?

A. If the patient has early Hepatitis C I would not start him on any vitamins because it may be wrongly concluded that the nutrients made that patient sick. If they have chronic Hepatitis C, I see no reason to withhold nutrients including vitamin C and niacin.

Relapses and orthomolecular therapy

Putting setbacks and relapses in perspective

Recovering from schizophrenia is often difficult as not all the symptoms disappear at the same rate. Many patients hallucinate less and have fewer delusions as they start the recovery process but they may become more depressed. As they start to recover they become more aware of how sick they have been and this in itself may be discouraging. But when this situation is explained to them by an understanding physician, then patients feel encouraged to continue and eventually the depression and anxiety diminish.

Patients and their families have to be very patient especially at the beginning of treatment because very few note any significant change within the first two months of starting treatment unless one of their main symptoms came from food allergies and they were placed on the elimination diet.

We learn that there may be setbacks, relapses. This is true of almost every known disease. But a relapse does not mean the game is over. It means that treatment must be continued and applied even more vigorously.

Modern psychiatry believes, and acts on that belief that side effects are not very important compared to the danger of a relapse and readmission into hospital. They are not willing to give patients a chance to see if they can remain well without these drugs.

An example was a young adolescent woman I saw who had responded very well to haldol with few side effects. But her psychiatrist agreed to do a drug study on one of the new drugs and started her on that drug instead. Over the next six months she gained over 60 pounds. This ruined her life. She was terribly uncomfortable with her weight, her shape and the fact that she was so disfigured by the obesity-inducing property of that drug. At her tender age, weight was an important issue of her life. She pleaded with her doctor to go back onto the haldol but he refused. He retorted "Better fat and well than psychotic and thin." In fact she was fat, but she was even sicker than she had been before.

My philosophy is that the patient's health is primary. If they have caused incapacitating side effects, the drugs should be withdrawn or so altered that the side effects no longer keep patients sick. In my opinion, it is better to give patients the chance, if they wish to take it, of going off medication if it is done carefully even if there is a risk of a relapse, because such relapses are readily dealt with by resuming the medication. Even if they need a few days in hospital to stabilize, this is better and more ethical for the patient. It follows the Golden Rule of Medicine: Do The Patient No Harm.

Canadian provinces have laws which force patients to take medication and if they refuse to do so they are forced back into hospitals. This is contrary to Canada's Constitution as decreed by the Supreme Court of Canada in 2003, acting on a case in the Province of Ontario. I expect eventually a few more cases will be heard and all of Canada will be forced to respect the Constitution.

Relapses are very disappointing to patients and their families. Many factors will lead to relapse including the flu, prolonged stress or sleeplessness, serious trauma, going back on foods to which the patients is allergic, not following the program and so on. Patients may be delighted with their new state of health, and assume they are cured and can never get sick again. A few of my patients suffered two or three relapses before they finally accepted the fact that they had to follow the program forever and then they are able to do so diligently.

A major problem arises from the rejection of orthomolecular psychiatry by psychiatrists in hospitals. In medicine we are accustomed to relapses no matter what the disease. A person may recover from pneumonia and be well for several years and then have another attack. We do not condemn them for this. But we should intensify our efforts to get them well again. If they have to be admitted and find an unsympathetic doctor in charge who will not allow them to take their vitamins, they will suffer a more serious relapse.

Many patients are very enterprising and take the vitamins anyway. One of my young male patients wore large boots unlaced at the top. He carried his vitamin pills in his boots and kept on taking them as he had before admission. In other cases families visit regularly and feed the vitamins to their relatives. They are merely continuing with a program that benefited their family member and they do not want to interrupt it.

Orthomolecular treatment for other mental illnesses

Slowing down aging, preventing senility and treating strokes

Aging is the accumulation of the effects of stress which are psychosocial, physical and biochemical. Oxidative stress is considered one of the main factors in premature aging.

Aging is one of the most complicated processes and cannot be discussed simply and succinctly. Therefore in this brief report only those measures which have been helpful will be discussed.

The impact of stress was proven by one of many experiments that mankind has imposed on itself. At the beginning of World War II in 1939, Japanese troops were marching on Hong Kong. The British government in desperation asked Canada for help. About 2,000 Canadian troops were sent, able-bodied, but unprepared and untrained. Arriving in Hong Kong they were promptly captured by the Japanese and remained prisoners of war for 44 months. The Canadians, hereafter called "Hong Kong veterans," suffered from total malnutrition including a very low calorie diet and were deficient in all the nutrients. They suffered from beri beri, pellagra, scurvy, infectious diarrhea and other conditions as well as from the brutality and incarceration without hope.

After 44 months, 25 percent of the prisoners were dead and the remainder were nearly dead, having lost about one third of their body weight. On the way back to Canada in hospital ships they were fed and given the only vitamins then available, rice bran extracts. They regained their weight and appeared to regain their health but they remained sick thereafter. Their plight was eventually recognized by the Canadian government who gave them special pensions. They suffered from a very high death rate, from cardiovascular disease, from blindness, from psychiatric and neurological illness. One year in these camps aged them four years so that after nearly four years in prison they were released, functionally 16 years older.

One of these Hong Kong Veterans, George, who had been sent along as the soldiers' physical instructor, remained permanently sick. He suffered from chronic pain from arthritis, heat and cold intolerance, depression and anxiety. He could not lift his arms higher than his shoulder and it took a half hour of combined effort of his wife and himself to mobilize him each morning so he could go to work. Because of his chronic disease, he was given heavy doses of barbiturates at night to help him fall asleep and after he awakened in the morning heavy doses of amphetamines to keep him awake. Because of his anxiety he was admitted to a psychiatric ward for treatment. He came home more anxious than before. His veterans administration file was voluminous.

In 1960 he was in charge of a retirement home. A study of the effect of niacin on some of the people living there peaked his interest and under his own direction be began to take niacin, 1 g three times daily. Two weeks later he felt completely normal with his symptoms gone. He was so delighted he rushed to tell his doctor. His doctor told him that niacin was toxic to the liver. George replied "Do you mean that I might feel this good for the next ten years and suddenly drop dead." His doctor agreed that was the likely outcome. George replied "It will have been worth it." His doctor became an enthusiastic practitioner of niacin therapy and before he died had treated several hundred patients with no evidence of liver toxicity.

George eventually became Lieutenant Governor of Saskatchewan where he died in office. Following his recovery he persuaded many Hong Kong Veterans and American Ex POWs from the Far East camps to start niacin. Those that did recovered.

The total stress imposed upon these healthy men rapidly aged them but the effects were reversible when they were given optimum doses of niacin. Of course niacin can not be the only factor. They had also been deficient in almost all the nutrients that they needed. The correct treatment is niacin but it must also include all the other nutrients as well. Perhaps niacin prevents the decrease in length of the telomeres. The pyridine nucleotide system, of which niacin is one of the most important components, helps control oxidative stress.

Since niacin prevents premature aging it should also inhibit the development of Alzheimer's disease and other conditions such as repeated micro-strokes that are aging factors. This it does. A recent report from the Rush Institute for Healthy Aging and Center for Disease Control and Prevention, Atlanta, concluded "In this prospective study we observed a protective association of niacin against the development of Alzheimer's Disease and cognitive decline with normal levels of dietary intake, which could have substantial public health implications for disease prevention if confirmed in further research".

A report in Annals New York Academy of Science concluded that niacin-bound chromium (glucose tolerance factor contains niacin and chromium) combined with grape seed extract improved insulin sensitivity, decreased free radical formation and reduced the symptoms of chronic age-related disorders including syndrome X. High HDL protects against dementia according to the 15-year Women's Health Study, in which 4,081 women, aged 66 and older, were divided into five quintiles for HDL levels. The highest HDL group had 73 mg/dL and the lowest 36 mg/dL. The women in the highest quintile had five times less chance of having cognitive impairment. The only substance that consistently elevates HDL is niacin.

What happened to an identical twin pair of women is very instructive. Identical twins are ideal for comparison controlled trials. In animal studies it is recognized that one identical twin pair is equivalent to two groups containing 40 non-related animals. One twin developed fast-onset Alzheimer's and died within a few years. Her identical twin sister then started on a comprehensive megavitamin program. She lived another 30 years mentally normal and then died of a stroke.

Dr. Roger Williams died when he was 95 years of age. He discovered folic acid and pantothenic acid. Toward the end of his life he was nearly totally deaf and blind but his mind was as sharp as ever. He still attended meetings and was with us in London in 1971 when we presented our findings about orthomolecular psychiatry and helped start the schizophrenia group in Great Britain. Dr. Williams told me that he was so sorry he had not started taking the vitamins early enough. He was sure he would have prevented these two major infirmities.

One of my female patients is 111 years old, alive and well both physically and mentally. At age 111, as the oldest person in Saskatchewan, she was still cross-country skiing. She has been on niacin for 41 years. The world's oldest human was 116 last year in Russia. Maybe the Saskatchewan patient will soon have the world's record. In December, 2004, I received the following note from her son: "There is one person older in Canada, but only our entry has all her wits about her and can walk. Seriously, she has always said that she followed the Hoffer program. There is a three-page spread on her in a Saskatchewan paper showing her skiing, rafting and horseback riding."

At our annual international Nutritional Medicine Today Conference in 2004 we announced the first members of the new Orthomolecular Medicine Hall of Fame. Listed below are the members, their age span (mean 84) and their main area of nutritional interest. Unlike most people, their productivity did not decrease, but increased with age. The vitamins they studied and promoted are also given in the following table.

Linus Pauling, 1901–1994
Vitamin C

William. McCormick, 1880–1968
Vitamin C

Roger Williams, 1893–1988
Folate, pantothenate

Wilfrid Shute, 1907–1982
Vitamin E

Evan Shute, 1905–1978
Vitamin E

Irwin Stone, 1907–1984
Vitamin C

Carl Pfeiffer, 1908–1988
Vitamins B and C

Allan Cott, 1910–1993
Niacin

William Kaufman, 1910–2000
Nicotinamide

Humphry Osmond, 1917–2004
Niacin and C

Alzheimer's disease

In *What Really Causes Alzheimer's Disease*, Harold D. Foster writes "It has been know for over a century that aluminum is a neurotoxin. The unfortunate truth that its widespread use, by calcium and magnesium deficient populations, is the major cause of Alzheimer's disease is now unavoidable." Many factors are discussed in this valuable book. The solution is simple: eliminate aluminum from our food and environment and increase calcium and magnesium

The main B vitamin is niacin. But other nutrients are involved including other B vitamins, vitamin E and C which taken together decrease the incidence of Alzheimer's Disease. Dr. Peter Zandi, Johns Hopkins School of Public Health, said that "Vitamin E and C may offer protection against Alzheimer's disease when taken together in the higher doses available from individual supplements." They decreased the risk by 78%. Essential minerals such as selenium and zinc are important as they counteract the accumulation of toxic metals such as aluminum and mercury. Essential fatty acids play a major role. In short, optimal nutrition will be the most decisive factor in slowing down the ravages of aging.

Niacin may inhibit the development of Alzheimer's disease but unfortunately I have not found it helpful in treating the condition once it has been established. However about one third of all patents diagnosed Alzheimer's disease will at autopsy, not show the typical pathological findings. The clinical syndrome is the same but the causes are different. I suspect that these patients are more apt to have had a series of small strokes. In these cases, niacin will be more helpful. Alzheimer's patients most often have elevated cholesterol levels suggesting that cerebrovascular senile patients will more often have Alzheimer's disease.

Stroke

Each year about 500,000 people in the United States have their first stroke and 100,000 have a recurrent stroke. About 25% die each year after their first stroke. Niacin by correcting lipid profiles reduces one of the risk factors, perhaps the most important one.

I studied the effect of niacin on patients who had been brain damaged by stroke or by trauma. I became interested after reading a report from Sweden many years ago about the treatment of strokes, The authors reported that stroke patients on admission to hospital were promptly given IV niacin and that there was marked reduction in the incidence of stroke sequelae. After that a number of patients were referred to me having had a stroke or brain trauma. One was a middle-aged woman who had prided herself on her memory. She had a mild stroke but after her recovery her memory was not nearly as good and she found this a terrible handicap. After a few months on niacin, her memory was partially restored.

Another case was a young man who had a heavy object fall on his head in an industrial accident. After two years he was able to talk and to walk with a limp but he had not regained his interest in reading. Before that he had been an avid reader. After three months on niacin he regained some of his interest. It is possible that niacin, by dilating the capillaries, accelerated healing and increased the ability of the brain tissue to repair itself.

The addictions

Ideally, addicted patients should be off the substances to which they are addicted it but in most cases this is impossible and in all cases it is very difficult to achieve. The introduction of orthomolecular therapy to Alcoholics Anonymous by its co-founder, Bill W., was a great boon to alcoholics wanting to recover from this addiction. But even with AA it is rare that more than one third of the patients are able to remain off their addicting alcohol and drugs. Bill W always insisted that in addition to Alcoholics Anonymous members should also have any psychiatric problems treated.

There are two phases in the treatment (1) To help the patients get off the drugs and (2) To treat them so that they are comfortable off these drugs. To establish sobriety, the most helpful organization is AA and the offshoot groups available as social services in urban centers. If the addict has joined any of these groups, treatment is much more successful.

However, they may still remain very uncomfortable, with feelings of being very tense, anxious or depressed. This may strongly indicate that they may be suffering from depression or other mental disorders. These must be treated as described earlier. For alcoholics the most effective treatment is niacin in doses up to 1 g three times daily. Bill W. recognized this early and the information was distributed to physicians who are also members of AA and have their own medical association. A few treatment centers combining the principles of AA and orthomolecular psychiatry are reporting up to 80% recovery rates.

Learning and behavioral disorders

The same therapeutic principles apply to children as to adults. Diagnosis can be very simple. They should be examined for the usual possible problems such as organic brain damage, epilepsy, rare genetic abnormalities, for autism and for childhood schizophrenia. But for the broad group of children who are the ADHD and ADD children and include any type of learning and/or behaviour disorder, descriptive diagnosis is of little value in determining treatment.

Diagnosis should be etiologic and not descriptive. For children with learning and/or behavioral disorders, the first investigation must include examination for food allergies. The common ones are dairy products and sugar. These problems are rarer in children who have been breast-fed but they too can be allergic to the same foods. Most often they are allergic to formula, milk and sugar, infant food. Then one should try an elimination diet to ensure that the right foods are identified.

Children hate to give up sugar but if they are shown how harmful it is, they will cooperate. One of the ways is the junk Saturday routine. The child agrees to give up sugar and any suspect food from Monday to Friday. But on Saturday he is given all the junk and food he is allergic to. This will usually make him very sick. Sunday is recovery day and he resumes his program again until the child demands that he/she will no longer eat junk food.

For physicians just starting out only one vitamin may be necessary. Niacinamide is preferred because children do not like the niacin flush. But niacinamide is best given in capsules as it is very bitter. The usual starting dose is 500 mg three times daily after meals.

Vitamin C is helpful but not nearly as important. The usual dose is 1 to 3 g daily. Until the physician is familiar with these two vitamins, there is no need to add any more. But many children do have the signs of pyroluria and they will benefit from the addition of B6 up to 250 mg daily after meals and zinc ranging from 15 to 50 mg daily. The most commonly observed signs (of zinc and pyridoxine deficiency) are white areas in the finger nails, stria in the skin, sore knees, pale complexion and of course learning and behaviour disorders. Ideally, the child should be urine-tested for the mauve factor.

If the child is already on Ritalin or other sympathomimetic drugs, the orthomolecular program must be given a chance to work, which could take up to 6 months before attempts are made to reduce the drugs. Parents will usually know when to stop the medication. With this simple approach, the majority of children will recover.

Starting in 1960 I have treated well over 2,000 patients under the age of 14 (Hoffer, 2004) There were very few failures and when they did occur it was often because the parents were not able to supervise their children's programs effectively. Often one or both parents are also ill and should be treated. Schizophrenic children respond very well. In 1960 a young couple with 4 children were expelled from the town in which they were living because both parents were so psychotic the city could not deal with them and threatened to commit them to the closest mental hospital. They fled to Saskatoon and were given orthomolecular treatment. The father was well in a few months and has been well since and working full time. The mother went to university, received an MA and is now a senior administrator. Of their four children, three showed signs of behavioral problems. With these children, dairy products were eliminated, they were given vitamins, and today the entire family is normal.

Reference

Hoffer, A., (2004). Healing Children's Attention & Behavior Disorders. CCNM Press, Toronto.

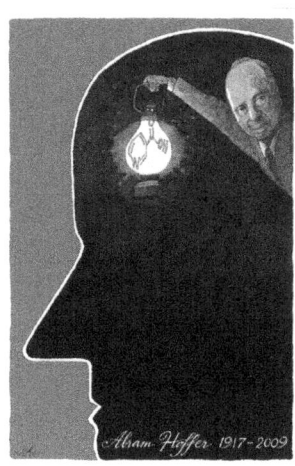

Conclusion

Schizophrenia is a complicated condition that is often not well addressed by conventional medicine and psychiatry. Dr. Hoffer's work opened the door to recognizing biochemical promoters and drivers of schizophrenia.

This update presents research and information acquired since Dr. Hoffer's passing in 2009, especially regarding the roles of poor diet, nutrient deficiencies, toxins, and metabolic conditions. With this knowledge comes the potential for better answers, better solutions, and hope for people with schizophrenia and clinicians.

Biographies

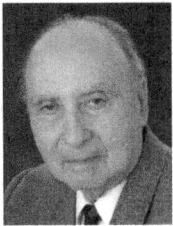

Abram Hoffer, MD, PhD

Dr. Abram Hoffer dedicated his career to discovering and sharing the biochemical drivers of mental health symptoms. Over the span of his career he helped thousands of patients, and educated doctors and families, on how to use nutrients to effectively address schizophrenia.

Abram Hoffer, was born in 1917 in Canada on a southern Saskatchewan farm. Raised on the land, he developed an ethic for hard work, perseverance, humility, honesty, and caring for others. In high school, he developed a passion that would be central to his life work—chemistry. Abram chose Agricultural Chemistry for his Masters degree as a compromise between his fathers wish that he stay on the farm, and his wish to continue his education. In 1944, Abram received his PhD in biochemistry from University of Minnesota, where he learned about the importance and roles of B-vitamins.

Abram was hired by Purity Flour Mills in Winnipeg in 1941 to measure the amount of thiamine (vitamin B1) being added to the flour as part of the enrichment process. The enriching of flour was implemented by the Canadian government to address the effects of nutrient deficiencies in Canadian and British solders during World War II. Abram, grateful for the opportunity, enthusiastically set up the lab and necessary procedures, but found maintaining the lab unfulfilling, and after four years, resigned.

Unsure of what to do next, Abram followed his wife Rose's suggestion to become a medical doctor, with his preclinical studies at the University of Saskatoon, completing his courses and medical exams at University of Toronto, and his Internship at Saskatoon City Hospital.

Abram had intended to go into general practice, but instead developed an interest in psychiatry, and as a result, in 1950 he accepted three concurrent jobs in the psychiatric wing of Regina's General Hospital, a psychiatric resident (in order to learn psychiatry), a biochemistry consultant for the pathology department, and Director of Psychiatric Research.

The experience Abram gained from these positions ultimately gave him clarity about what he wanted, which was to integrate his knowledge of chemistry, medicine, and psychiatry to pursue a career in psychiatric research. The idea was especially attractive because, at the time very little was known about useful mental health treatments.

Over the years that followed, Abram collaborated with his contemporaries to expand understanding in the field of orthomolecular psychiatry, making significant contributions to mental health knowledge and treatments.

Accomplishments Abram was associated with include:
- the discovery of the importance and roles of niacin and vitamin C in schizophrenia,
- developing the adrenochrome hypothesis, the first biochemical theory to explain schizophrenia,
- establishing the kryptopyrrole theory in regards to schizophrenia
- implementing the first nutritional schizophrenia treatments, which doubled recovery rates, and started the field of Orthomolecular Psychiatry,
- running the first ever double-blind trials in psychiatry, and
- discovering that niacin lowers cholesterol, giving birth to the new paradigm of "vitamins as treatment".

As Abram and his colleagues shared their research and findings, they faced relentless politically-driven rejection from establishment organizations intent on keeping the status quo. In spite of this, Abram persevered, deciding it was more important to help his schizophrenic patients than to "please the psychiatric profession".

Abram's lifetime efforts to promote the nutrient based approach to helping schizophrenia patients included:
- writing over two dozen books and over 500 papers, as well as co-authoring books and papers with Linus Pauling and Humphrey Osmond;
- leading the American Schizophrenia Association, the Canadian Schizophrenia Foundation, and the International Schizophrenia Foundation;
- founding the International Society for Orthomolecular Medicine; and
- a 42-year tenure as Co-Editor and Editor in chief for the *Journal of Orthomolecular Medicine* (originally the *Journal of Schizophrenia*, and *Journal of Orthomolecular Psychiatry*).

Abram started a private practice in 1967. He continued helping patients for 38 years, utilizing diet, nutrients, as well as standard psychiatric therapies. In addition to treating thousands of schizophrenia and other mental health patients, he also treated over 1,300 cancer patients using the orthomolecular approach.

Dr. Abram Hoffer is remembered for his sense of humour, his deep caring for the plight of his patients, and his willingness to find and share useful solutions for people suffering from schizophrenia. His legacy lives on in the many people and organizations who continue to explore, expand, and use the "nutrients as medicine" approach for addressing mental health.

Books written by Dr. Hoffer include:

Hoffer A. *Niacin Therapy in Psychiatry*. CC Thomas, Springfield, IL (1962)

Hoffer A & Osmond H. *How to Live With Schizophrenia*. University Books, New York, NY, 1966. Also published by Johnson, London, 1966. Written with Fannie Kahan. New and Revised Ed. Citadel Press, New York, NY, 1992. Revised Ed. Quarry Press, Kingston, ON (1999)

Kelm H, Hoffer A & Osmond H. *Hoffer-Osmond Diagnostic Manual*. Saskatoon, SK (1967)

Hoffer A. *The Hallucinogens*. Academic Press (1967)

Hoffer A, Kelm H & Osmond H. *The Hoffer-Osmond Diagnostic Test*. RE Krieger Pub. Co., Huntington, NY (1975)

Hoffer A. *Megavitamin therapy: In reply to the American Psychiatric Association Task Force Report on Megavitamins and Orthomolecular Psychiatry*. Canadian Schizophrenia Foundation (1976)

Hoffer A. *Dr Abram Hoffer's Guide to the Identification and Treatment of Schizophrenia*. Keats Pub (1980)

Hoffer A & Walker M: *Nutrients to Age Without Senility*. Keats Pub Inc, New Canaan, CT (1980)

Hoffer A. *Vitamin B3 (Niacin)*. McFarland & Company (1982)

Hoffer A. *Common Questions on Schizophrenia and their Answers*. Keats Pub (1987)

Hoffer A. *Nutrition for the General Practitioner*. Keats Pub (1988)

Hoffer A. *Orthomolecular Medicine for Physicians*. Keats Pub., New Canaan, CT (1989)

Hoffer A. *Vitamin B-3 and Schizophrenia. Discovery, Recovery, Controversy*. Quarry Press, Kingston, ON (1999)

Hoffer A. *Common Questions on Schizophrenia and Their Answers*. Keats Pub, New Canaan, CT, 1988. Reprinted Quarry Press, Kingston, ON (1999)

Hoffer A, Walker M. *Putting It All Together: The New Orthomolecular Nutrition*. Keats Publishing Inc. New Canaan, Conn, 1996. Also: McGraw-Hill (1998)

Hoffer A. Hoffer's *A.B.C. of Natural Nutrition for Children*. Quarry Press. Kingston, ON (1999)

Hoffer A. *Orthomolecular Treatment for Schizophrenia*. Keats, Lincolnwood, Ill (1999)

Hoffer A. *Vitamin C and Cancer: Discovery, Recovery, Controversy*. Quarry Press, Kingston, ON (2000)

Hoffer A, Walker M: *Smart Nutrients: Prevent and Treat Alzheimer's, Enhance Brain Function*. Vital Health Publishing; 2nd Rev edition (2002)

Hoffer A. *Healing Schizophrenia. Complementary Vitamin & Drug Treatments*. CCNM Press (2004)

Hoffer A. *Healing Children's Attention & Behavior Disorders: Complementary Nutritional & Psychological Treatments.* CCNM Press (2004)

Hoffer A, Pauling L. *Healing Cancer: Complimentary Vitamin & Drug Treatments.* CCNM Press (2004)

Hoffer A. *Adventures in Psychiatry: The Scientific Memoirs of Dr. Abram Hoffer.* Caledon, Ontario: KOS Publishing (2005)

Hoffer A, Prousky J. *Naturopathic Nutrition: A Guide to Nutrient-rich Food & Nutritional Supplements for Optimum Health.* CCNM Press (2006)

Hoffer A, Foster HD. *Feel Better, Live Longer With Vitamin B-3: Nutrient Deficiency and Dependency.* CCNM Press (2007)

Dr. James Greenblatt, MD
Medical Director, Psychiatry Redefined, Chief Medical Officer, Walden Behavioral Care

A pioneer in the field of integrative medicine, James M. Greenblatt, MD has treated patients with complex behavioral and mood disorders since 1990. After receiving his medical degree from George Washington University School of Medicine, Dr. Greenblatt completed his psychiatry residency at George Washington University Medical Center.

Dr. Greenblatt completed a two-year fellowship at Johns Hopkins University School of Medicine, became board certified in child and adolescent psychiatry, and served as Chief Resident.

During the fellowship, Dr. Greenblatt received specialized training in the diagnosis and treatment of disorders that appear in childhood, such as attention deficit hyperactivity disorder (ADHD), behavioral disorders, autism spectrum disorders, and complex mood and anxiety disorders.

Dr. Greenblatt developed an outpatient clinic, Comprehensive Psychiatric Resources, to address biochemical individuality and the underlying biological mechanisms that may contribute to or cause psychiatric symptoms. The clinic provided patient-centered care for families with children struggling with ADHD and other behavioral disorders.

Dr. Greenblatt's expertise in integrative medicine attracted patients from all across the world seeking consultations for complex mood, behavioral, and eating disorders.

For the last three decades, Dr. Greenblatt has devoted his career to educating his colleagues, clinicians, and patients how integrative medicine can have profound effects on mental wellness and how to employ balanced, integrative strategies in the treatment mental illness.

Dr. Greenblatt currently serves as the Chief Medical Officer at Walden Behavioral Care in Waltham, MA and serves as an Assistant Clinical Professor of Psychiatry at Tufts University School of Medicine and Dartmouth College Geisel School of Medicine.

Dr. Greenblatt was inducted into the Orthomolecular Medicine Hall of Fame in 2017.

Books written by Dr. Greenblatt include:

Finally Focused: The Breakthrough Natural Treatment Plan for ADHD That Restores Attention, Minimizes Hyperactivity, and Helps Eliminate Drug Side Effects (2017)

Nutritional Lithium: The Cinderella Story (2016)

Integrative Therapies for Depression: Redefining Models for Assessment, Treatment, and Prevention (2015)

Answers to Binge Eating (2014)

The Breakthrough Depression Solution (2012)

Answers to Anorexia (2011)

Dr. Jonathan Prousky, ND, MSc, MA
Chief Naturopathic Medical Officer, Professor, Canadian College of Naturopathic Medicine

Dr. Jonathan Prousky received his undergraduate degree from the University of Toronto (physical and health education), and his N.D. (naturopathic doctor) degree from Bastyr University. He also obtained Masters degrees from the University of London (primary health care) and Yorkville University (counselling psychology).

Dr. Prousky has been in private practice for more than two decades, and has primarily focused his clinical practice on the evaluation and management of mental health, with integrative orthomolecular and botanical (plant-based) medicines.

Dr. Prousky is the current Chief Naturopathic Medical Officer at the Canadian College of Naturopathic Medicine (Toronto, Canada), and has been employed at the college since 2000. While his primary role is to oversee the health care provided to patients, and monitor best practices and the medical procedures used at the college and the college's clinics, he has been a spirited lecturer, professor, and mentor to many students and interns for more than 20 years.

In 2009 Dr. Prousky served as the spokesperson for the Canada-wide Orthomolecular Health Campaign, giving dozens of television, radio and print interviews and participating in other publicity engagements. With the Canadian Society for Orthomolecular Medicine, he presented several medical seminars in orthomolecular treatment for mental disorders. He has lectured extensively on mental health and other topics throughout North America to medical doctors, naturopathic doctors, other health care providers, and patients.

Following the death of Dr. Abram Hoffer, Dr. Prousky assumed the editorship of the *Journal of Orthomolecular Medicine*. He was the first naturopathic doctor to receive the "Orthomolecular Doctor of the Year" award in 2010, and was inducted into the Orthomolecular Medicine Hall of Fame in 2017.

Dr. Prousky has over 50 publications in peer reviewed medical journals from the complementary and alternative discipline.

Books written by Dr. Prousky include:

Anxiety: Orthomolecular Diagnosis and Treatment (2006)

Naturopathic Nutrition (2006)

Hoffer & Prousky on Anxiety (2009)

The Vitamin Cure for Chronic Fatigue Syndrome (2010),

The Textbook of Integrative Clinical Nutrition (2012)

Paul Demeda, CNP

Paul Demeda has empowered people to consciously and holistically manage their health for over 15 years. He is dedicated to investigating, clarifying, and explaining important nutrition issues and concepts, and is an ardent proponent of critical thinking in the context of health, and published research.

Paul graduated from York University in Toronto in 1984 and earned his diploma in Applied Holistic Nutrition from The Institute of Holistic Nutrition in 2004. He became an fervent advocate for Orthomolecular Medicine as a result of attending the 2009 Orthomolecular Medicine Today conference.

Paul taught clinical nutrition courses for 16 years, and created nutrition courses for Institute of Holistic Nutrition, Centennial College in Toronto, and the Edison Institute of Nutrition. He lectures on a range of health topics including mental health, detoxification, and critical thinking, and presented at the 43rd and 47th International Orthomolecular Medicine Today conferences in Vancouver.

Paul maintains clinical practice at the D'Avignon Digestive Health Centre and the Wellness Institute in Toronto, where he specializes in the areas of digestive issues, mental health, and cancer. Paul is Program Facilitator at the International Society for Orthomolecular Medicine.

Acknowledgements

In publishing this timely, important update to Abram Hoffer's 2007 book, *Orthomolecular Treatment for Schizophrenia*, we are especially grateful to our friends and colleagues, James Greenblatt and Jonathan Prousky. The new chapters and material gleaned from their seminars and articles demonstrate their deep commitment to and knowledge of orthomolecular medicine. Their decades of experience provide superb support and enhancement to Abram's work in schizophrenia.

We are fortunate that Paul Demeda took on the formidable task of melding Abram's original text with new materials and references. More than the book's editor, Paul served as its dedicated, meticulous and skillful amalgamator to produce this new volume.

Thanks also go to Steven Carter, editor/publisher of the first edition of this book, who worked with Abram for 22 years at the *Journal of Orthomolecular Medicine* and as the Executive Director of the International Schizophrenia Foundation; to Frances Fuller, Abram's assistant, collaborator and business associate of 32 years; and to Andrew Cuscianna for overseeing this project and for his valuable support.

We are most grateful for the generous donation that has made this republication of Abram Hoffer's work possible for today's readership.

Finally, we continue to honour and respect the enormous contribution that Abram Hoffer made to those with schizophrenia; his generosity and intelligence continue to bring light to mental illness through his pioneering works in orthomolecular medicine.

The Board of Directors
International Society for Orthomolecular Medicine

Made in United States
Orlando, FL
25 August 2022